To be effective, the yoga postures (asanas) described and illustrated in this book require a musical elixir. The elixirs are included with purchase of the book. To obtain your copy of this music, you may:

A. To download the music, go to: www.yogaofillumination.com

B. For the physical CD
   a. email sj@almine.net and provide your name, mailing address and phone number.

   b. call toll-free 877 552-5646 or 614 354-2071

The elixirs work in conjunction with the postures, using the alchemical potencies of frequency incorporated within the music.

Many blessings, dearest. May the future unfold before you in passion and joy, with love, Almine

SARADESI SATVA YOGA

The Yoga of Eternal Youth

Almine

Practical Wisdom for Spiritual
Mastery

Published by Spiritual Journeys LLC

Copyright 2011 MAB 998 Megatrust

By Almine
Spiritual Journeys LLC
P.O. Box 300
Newport, Oregon 97365

Cover Layout by Rogier Chardet

Cover Art by Dorian Dyer
Website: visionheartart.com
Contributing artist: Eva Pulnicki

Modeling by Jaylene

www.spiritualjourneys.com
Toll-free number 877 552-5646

ISBN 978-1-936926-05-3 (Softcover)
ISBN 978-1-936926-04-6 (Adobe Reader)

Contents

About the Author.. IX

Introduction 1

The 144 Core Concepts of Separation 3

The Saradesi Satva Yoga Postures 83

Appendix I Notes for Teachers 113

Appendix II Disclaimer..115

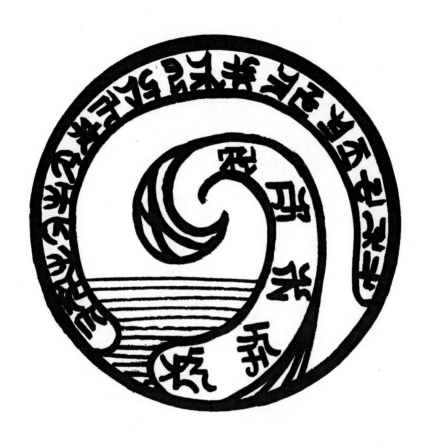

Kia-shatach
Saradesi Labyrinth of Renewal

ENDORSEMENTS

"What a priceless experience to be able to catch a glimpse into one of the most remarkable lives of our time ..."

H.E. Ambassador Armen Sarkissian
Former Prime Minister of the Republic of Armenia
Astro-physicist, Cambridge University, U.K.

****

"I'm really impressed with Almine and the integrity of her revelations. My respect for her is immense and I hope that others will find as much value in her teachings as I have."

Dr. Fred Bell
Former NASA Scientist

****

"The information she delivers to humanity is of the highest clarity. She is fully deserving of her reputation as the leading mystic of our age."

Zbigniew Ostas, Ph.D.
Quantum Medicine, Somatidian Orthobiology
Canada and Poland

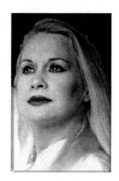

About the Author

Almine is a mystic, healer and teacher who traveled for years through many countries, empowering thousands of individuals who were drawn to her comprehensible delivery of advanced metaphysical concepts. In the wake of her humility and selfless service, unspeakable miracles have followed.

In her life, made rich by the mystical and the holy, she has stood face-to-face with many of the ancient Masters of light, retaining full memory of the ancient holy languages in both written and spoken form.

Her teachings are centered on the idea that it is not only possible to live a life of mastery and love, but that it is the birthright of every human to attain such levels of perfection. Her journey has become one of learning to live in the physical, maintaining the delicate balance of remaining self-aware while being fully expanded.

"When we live in the moment, we live in the place of power, aligned with eternal time and the intent of the Infinite. Our will becomes blended with that of the Divine."

— Almine

Saradesi Satva Yoga

THE YOGA OF ETERNAL YOUTH

As translated from the ancient texts of Saradesi—The Fountain of Youth

The ancient texts speak of time as movement. They affirm that time and space, movement and stillness, are illusions. To sustain any illusion requires an enormous amount of resources. This depletion of resources causes aging and decay.

The illusion of polarity, the impossibility that the One Life can be divided and split is brought to resolution by balancing the opposite poles exactly. Only then can they cancel one another out, revealing an incorruptible reality that lies beyond—the reality of Eternal Youth.

144 Core Illusions of Separation

Illumination 1

Illusion comes from an absence of light. To find the source of illusion, seek the understanding that is missing.

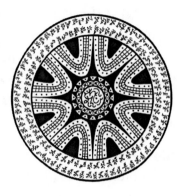

Exploitation comes from a misplaced desire for order. The mind perceives order as the compartmentalizing of life, the separating of oneness for the purpose of controlling through definition.

True order is the never-ending spontaneous flow of perfection of the One Life. Compartmentalization is duality. The nature of mind has been separative, to try to map out the incomprehensible. Those that seek to exploit are acting out the need of mind to create boundaries, by forcing others to do so.

By illuminating the recognition of the oneness of life, the true inclusive nature of mind assumes its place on the thrones of our lives. We live the truth that there is no relationship, there is only One Life.

Illumination 2

Mind can only decide whether an action is worth taking based upon assessment of past experience. Time as linear is an illusion. The past does not exist as real; all there is, is the fluid eternal moment. Because life changes in an exponential way as the fluid moment flows, linear predictability of outcome is impossible.

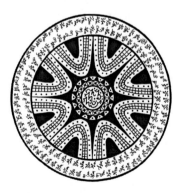

The addiction of mind to 'know' prevents us from allowing the spontaneous explosion of life's possibilities, keeping us in bondage to the mediocrity of the past. Addiction arises from self-abandonment. Mind abandons its inner knowingness by trying to understand itself through looking for answers without.

The illusion of without and within space disappears when truth is illuminated. That which appears to be without is part of us as well; the only reason anything can speak to us is because it is us speaking to ourselves.

Illumination 3

The gullible tendency of man to blindly follow arises from an inner prompting to receive and comply with the will of the Infinite. Creation was made to express the Divine Intent, to listen to the promptings of the Infinite's unfolding of new potential for expression.

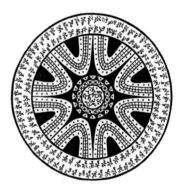

When the tyranny of mind replaced the soft whispers of the Divine, the deep-seated knowingness that free will is an illusion remained, leaving an information vacuum. This was a vulnerability that led us to take guidance from anyone who, with great conviction, could override our objections by convincing us that they know and we don't. The more sensitive we are, the more acutely we are aware that we don't know.

The illumination that life is an experience, not a set of guidelines to live by, needs to replace the need to know. Knowing consists of prison bars.

Illumination 4

Few are able to take responsibility for their own actions. Resources are expended without the guidance and understanding of the heart's motives. The creation of the illusion of intelligence, formed by mind to differentiate between the compartments it had created, contributes to this. Intelligence chooses between one thing and another. It 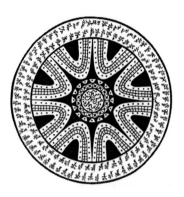 labels one thing as good and another as less so, leading to the origin of value judgments, as well as those of guilt and innocence.

It is under the labels of guilt and innocence that the motives for our actions hide. The mind's labeling is not flexible. It stereotypes and imprisons just as surely as any jailer, and gaining freedom is not easily accomplished.

When life is the expression of the One and mind has merged into the inclusive eternal mind that embraces rather than divides, there is no guilt. There can be no guilt when there is no choice, for we have become blended with the Will of the Infinite.

Illumination 5

Heroism and martyrdom have been extolled within individuated life. They are nevertheless illusions. How can one part of the ocean sacrifice itself for another part of the ocean, when the ocean is indivisible and incorruptible? Even if it could be so, would taking from one part to give to another not change the whole?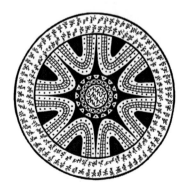

And if heroism consists in taking bold action in the face of a perceived threat, let us examine this illusion also. The person in oneness and vision sees the highest choice at all times: that which most fully reflects who we are, the one vast being having a human experience. In seeing it, we have no choice. To live less than our highest vision is un-impeccable. It is said: "Fortune favors the brave." The reason for this is that all of life supports one who lives in his highest truth; one who knows he is all that is.

Illumination 6

Responsibility can be carried like an identity, designating someone as being able to be counted on. The arrogance of thinking that we are needed in the ever-changing fluid patterns of life—that the smooth unfolding of life around us depends upon our contribution—is a fallacy.

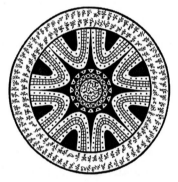

We do what is placed before us in the moment, with a great sense of adventure, for it is the doorway to the unfolding of life. When confronted with a choice, we gauge its validity by the joy it may bring, confident in the fact that our selection is already known and that life has already conformed around the outcome in a pattern of perfection.

We are not responsible for carrying life. Instead, it is cradling us in a cherished embrace.

Illumination 7

The inclination to be a 'respecter' of people, to value one above another, is remnant of the value judgments of intelligence created by separative mind. This illusion has held the masterful life of grace hostage and personal empowerment in a stranglehold. Few are exempt from its clutches.

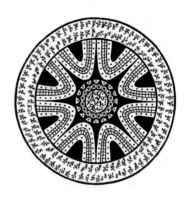

There is a flawed premise that if one has a child, it is to be expected that one would love that child more than other children. This depends upon how 'more' is defined. If it means that the degree to which other children are loved is less, we do not see the One Life running through all children. If it means there are more opportunities to see the wonder of life through the child you can watch grow from birth to adulthood, it is simply like looking through one window rather than another.

Illumination 8

Much effort is expended endeavoring to change our perspective to a higher one, to raise our perception. When all things are known to us and it is simply a matter of accessing such information, to what are we raising our perspective? There are no such things as accidents, nor is there anything in the cosmos to fix. If there is an 'occlusion' on any given moment in our perception, it is to guide us in a direction of

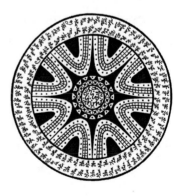

Infinite intent, like a pathway that becomes illuminated by dimming the surrounding forest.

7

The highest or best perception we can have for guidance in any moment is exactly the one we have. If there are portions of our vision dimmed, it is so the path can be more clearly indicated. This applies to others as well. We should remember this, as they make choices that appear flawed to us. There are no flawed choices. There is only the path along which we are led to perfection.

Illumination 9

Humor does not belong only to humankind. If we could understand, we could see that animals laugh too. Crows play pranks on one another. Animals and plants laugh when tickled by bees. Yet the accessing of the holy is viewed as a solemn affair—laughter at such times viewed as inappropriate. Self-appointed spi-

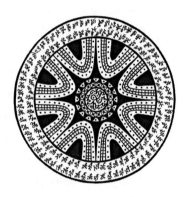

ritual leaders put on solemn faces to indicate how much in touch with the Divine they are.

Cosmic bliss is the movement of the Being of the Infinite. When a person experiences bliss, it is because to some extent the movement of the Infinite is felt within the cells—something more easily available when the cellular nucleus enlarges during mastery.

Humor is the holy experience of momentarily entering into the bliss of cosmic movement. Laughter is the release of such an overwhelmingly large experience. We enter the holy of holies through humor and it leaves us euphoric.

Illumination 10

Many have sought to remove density within life, wanting all to be illumina- ted. Great patterns of moving light of various gradations dance spontaneous- ly within existence. Changing areas of existence through varying shades of light is an exuberant expression of the Infinite's joy in beingness.

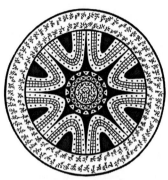

Density is nothing more than the areas of light that are slightly dimmed, without which there can be no pattern. It is the note that is not played as it waits its turn to add to the exquisite symphony of life. If all notes are played at once, there can be no music. If all light shines equally bright, there can be no definitions and no pattern.

Density, if it means that which does not belong, does not exist. If it means the deliberate withholding of the starburst of light each be- ing is, so that they may contribute to the perfection of life unfolding, it does and should exist.

Illumination 11

Authority is a structure of illusion, based on the selfappointed authority of mind. Authority in the form of external government cannot exist because rela- tionship, the premise upon which it is based, does not exist. In accepting it or imposing it as real, we validate the unreal.

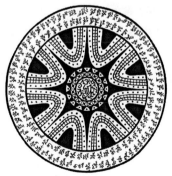

The only real government there is, is the self-government of the individual. The question may then be asked, if there is no freedom of choice, as we are enticed by our level of perception to participate in the cosmic dance, what we are governing?

We have the opportunity to gain insights into the self from the experience life leads us to. When we do, we contribute to the intricacy of the pattern of life, helping to shape the beauty of the dance. We are not needed to accomplish this, but rather are given the opportunity to share the joy.

Illumination 12

There is no real standard for beauty. The stem of the flower is not expected to appear as the bloom, nor the roots that languish in the cool depths of the soil to be like the leaves.

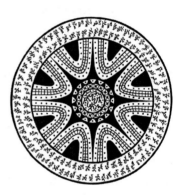

What makes the stem beautiful is the perfection with which it fulfills the purpose of its creation; the firmness with which it lifts the flower unto the sun; the pliant resilience with which it bends in the storm.

Each being has a specific part to play in the Being of the One Life. Each is uniquely beautiful in that beauty matches function. Yet none are locked into a specific function and, should life call for us to flow in another direction, we may. The aged may youthen and the care-worn become filled with lightness of being, yet the aged have no less beauty than the young.

Illumination 13

Conflict has existed among beings since the onset of individuated life. Yet in reality, there cannot be conflict. Because of this, there cannot be solutions either. What there can be is creative flow.

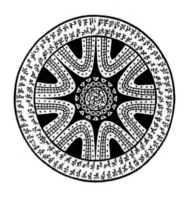

If the wild river, flowing freely and spontaneously, did not have its ever-altering obstacle course, its very nature would be compromised. It would no longer be a river, but a predictable canal. It is the newly fallen tree that alters the river's course that provides the spontaneous change in its shape.

Let us embrace the illumination that no two beings exist. All lives within us as part of the eternal symphony, orchestrated by the Infinite.

Illumination 14

Empathically resonating with the hardship of others can be an added perceived burden for those who are sensitive. When a note is played on a piano, careful observation will show every similar note in every octave vibrating in empathic resonance.

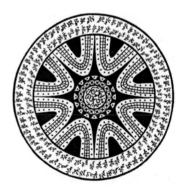

We only empathically resonate with what is already within our own lives, else we would not recognize, nor take on the emotions of another. The empath is therefore more sensitive than most in seeing the areas where illusion lingers, within their own perception causing distortion of emotion.

This too is in perfection. But when someone before us strikes a discordant note that resonates within us, it is time to move beyond it. We are not picking up someone else's debris—there is only one being: oneself.

Illumination 15

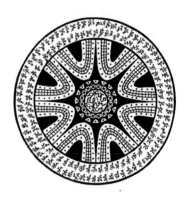

In the moment, we contain all that is. Overwhelm cannot exist because in the moment, infinite resources are accessed. It is when our workload is assessed linearly that we try to carry the accomplishments of many moments in the moment of the now. It is when work is seen in chunks that we cut ourselves off from cosmic resources and the load becomes heavy.

Are we overwhelmed by the grandeur of our vision? Of eternal joy flowing through our hearts? The outlets for such strong feelings that threaten to engulf us are laughter, song, tears, physical exercise or dance. The grandeur of the Infinite feels overwhelming only when we see ourselves as separate from It. The truth is that we are to dissolve ourselves into and become one with It.

Illumination 16

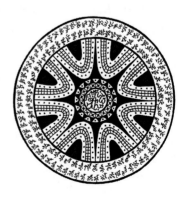

Power is released when a lower order changes to a higher order. For either order to exist implies that there are moments when the exuberant flow of Infinite life is contained and static, that a matrix can in reality exist and that life is less than spontaneous.

Power is not only the effect of change, but seen as necessary to effect change. What could we possibly want to change, if all beings are acting, not of their volition, but as part of the orchestrated perfection of the whole? If opposition is merely a signal from the One Life to change direction, how can it be seen as something to remove? In a cosmos of perfection, there is nothing to change; there is nothing for which power is needed. The One Life supports us.

Illumination 17

Comparison implies relationship and attempts to define something by what it is not. This type of definition mistakenly leads us to believe that we understand the essence of something because we can see what it is not. Yet this reveals nothing of what it is.

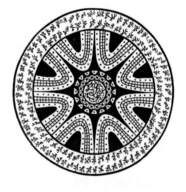

If comparison is done to determine value, we are using the old illusory tool of intelligence and imposing non-existent, past experiential knowledge and value systems on the newness of the moment.

There are times when the tiny tack is needed. There are times when the big bolt is exactly right. Each is perfect for a unique function.

There is no way we can determine value other than by what is applicable for this moment. Choices can only be deemed as accurate or not moment by moment, as life dances on its way.

Illumination 18

Energy is the result of the movement of something between two parts, or the dispersal of energy—the result of movement away from a point of origin.

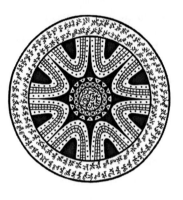

If we had freedom of choice, we would be in a separate space within the Infinite's Being. We would also be artificial intelligence and unreal. But as part of the limitless Being of One Life, we are real and no longer have a separate movement from the whole. We move as the Infinite moves, in limitless Oneness.

We have become directionless movement without points of origin or reference points. Like the ocean, we have become all resources and they no longer exist separate from us. Energy has no real existence.

Illumination 19

Life force has been defined as that which enlivens. It is inherent within the creation of the Infinite, rather than the artificial sub-creations of man. It is one of the building blocks of existence and, like all others, an illusion.

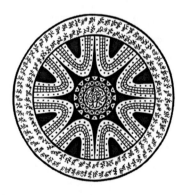

Does the table or the chair man has made truly exist? No, for within the One Life only one Self—Creator exists. In fluidity The Infinite self-creates moment by moment. There is no place for rigid structure and, as man sees through the illusions, the sub-creations will begin to disappear. The physical body will fluidly change moment by moment as we do. In spaceless space it is a fluid part of the dance, no longer a rigid reference point in the vastness of our Being.

Illumination 20

Life affirming joyousness of the Self is the quality of the true reality of life. There is no possibility that self-destructiveness can exist. Life dances in joyous innovation. There is no place for structure.

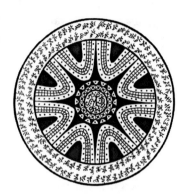

Attempts to create controlled structure bring stagnation, decay and self-destructiveness. These things are illusions.

When mind created structures, it also invented the concept that growth was necessary. This replaced the illusion of destructiveness with the illusion of the need to strive in order to grow. As programs to strive kept us from being self-destructive, we became trapped in their illusions and others, like linear becoming. There is only life spontaneously lived.

Illumination 21

Indulging an illusion as part of personality, or by letting it become identity, retains the illusion that we have that personality or identity. Personality either forms as a result of personal history or as a partial expression of all the traits of the One Life within us. In reality, there is no past, no memory of personal history. Everything lives

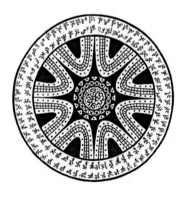

within us and can be expressed. Illusion bars us from full expression and illusion cannot exist within the One Life.

It is not 'holy' or 'enlightened' to cling to separation-based views. That does not serve life. Let all fractures be gone—let wholeness reign.

Illumination 22

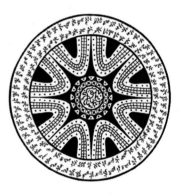

We have used suffering to stay contracted when we have encountered the limitless vastness of our being. Focusing on suffering allows us to avoid seeing our true self.

Suffering is an illusion born of the illusion that loss can occur, that we can be alone, that imperfection or injustice can exist within the perfection of One Being. We allow this even as the fullness of life moves through us.

But within the vastness of life, neither contraction nor expansion can exist because there is no direction, nor is there a focal point. We are all things, filling the vastness of existence with our unique presence.

Illumination 23

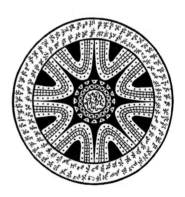

Seeing flaws in others occurs when we do not want to see the same flaw in our self. The judgment is inflexible once intelligence pronounces it. The self-censure this brings is painful because of the misplaced trust we have given to the self-appointed authority of the intellect. If we are irrevocably branded as bad or flawed, we believe we do not deserve good things in life.

The missing perception is that creations of the Infinite cannot be flawed. All beings play roles that form the kaleidoscope of changing life within the One Being. All are therefore innocent participants in the joyous pageantry of existence.

Illumination 24

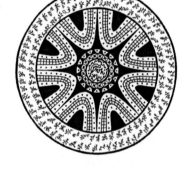

It is easier to see the support of the tribe than the support of the Oneness of Life. However, the individual cannot trust the illusion of relationship—in this case with the tribe—for support. The only support there is, is the self-support of the One Life.

The tribe traps with demands of conformity. It demands that the individual behave according to the tribe's ideas of what is normal; that bright lights be dimmed in exchange for the sense of false security which the tribe offers.

Instead we must adopt the absolute conviction that *our being is our sustenance,* and that the One Life of which we are an integral part, is our passage to freedom from ensnarement by the tribe's illusory promises of acceptance and support.

Illumination 25

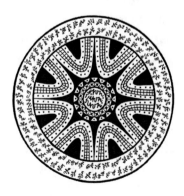

Disillusionment and disappointment when our ideals are not met and life around us seems much more unenlightened than we are, weighs heavily on the shoulders of lightworkers. Life seems inhospitable to the bright lights of the world.

The definition of the bright lights comes from the fact that the surrounding lights are dimmer. Every concerto has it crescendos and every dance it apex. Because we happen to be the apex of our surroundings does not mean the dance itself is mediocre, or that others may not yet surpass our brightness. Only the Grand Choreographer spontaneously delegates the roles.

Illumination 26

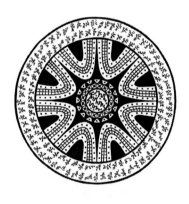

Complexity and simplicity cannot be viewed as having their own, individual realities. They are indivisibly connected, like two sides of one coin. As the cosmic symphony is playing, we can isolate and hear only the sound of the one note, middle C, as it is played every few bars. We would call this selective hearing of the one note 'simplicity'.

Alternatively, we could call the whole symphony complex, yet it is made up of single notes. In this way simplicity and complexity are both the result of an error of perception, or hearing. The whole is a spontaneous production that defies description as it changes each part of the fluid, eternal moment.

Illumination 27

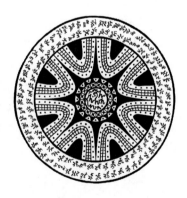

Life seems to require so much of us. Yet the only valid requirement is that we surrender to the One Life in which we exist, that we trust the benevolent support of That which gave us life. We were not created to suffer. Suffering is, after all, only an illusion. We were created to revel in the joy of living.

The self-imposed burdens of life have come through allowing the social conditioning and programs of others to govern us. When it is realized that we have forever as a being of immortality, the haste to accomplish certain things within a certain time frame ceases. We lay our burdens down and enjoy our work as part of the adventure.

Illumination 28

Expectations of duration are formed by the bondage of linear time. We assume from past experience that traveling or task or sleep require certain amounts of time. Because of our expectations, this illusion is perpetuated.

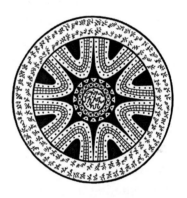

When we live in the timelessness of the One Life, the illusion of electromagnetics, which is part of duality, does not exist. It has been this illusion that has given the appearance of a delay between cause and effect. Eliminating clocks as much as we can, together with our flawed expectations of linear time, will set us free.

Illumination 29

We regard some people as fortunate and others as unfortunate. This illusion fails to recognize that every life is perfect within the grand design. A second illusion is that ease of living, as we perceive it, brings more joy or more fulfillment than a more arduous life.

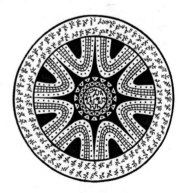

We so often do not see the pain of a fruitless life or one devoid of love and passion. The stress felt by a CEO driving an expensive car is less obvious than that of the person who must catch a fish for his next meal. In truth, the life of the latter may be far more satisfying, tranquil and lifeenhancing.

Illumination 30

Categorizing as holy and unholy or proper and improper comes from the judgments of the intellect. Using past conditioning as a gauge it attempts to control through labeling. Trying to fit our lives into categories diminishes more and more the spontaneity of our actions.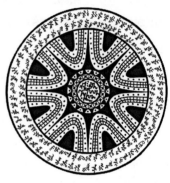

Those who live spontaneously, who are deemed 'wild and free' rather than 'civilized and responsible' are viewed with suspicion. The labeling is simply another form of programming by the tribe. The demeanor of those living freely and spontaneously could become contagious and control by the tribe could slip away. Man could instead break free into his natural state.

Illumination 31

Maturity is prized as a trait of leadership. Both these terms need to be examined as the illusions they are. Maturity carries the baggage of past programming and experiential knowledge. This closes the future to its new possibilities and denies the present its boundless exponential growth.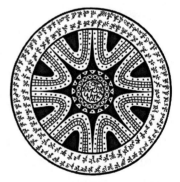

Because of the tendency of beings to follow authority, others are led around and around the fish bowl of the known in mediocrity. Leadership comes from certainty and conviction that the answers we have are valid. In every moment, the

One Life changes all previous possibilities. There is absolutely no valid basis for predictability—the hallmark of mediocrity.

Illumination 32

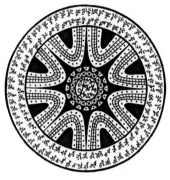

Damage from trauma is an illusion based on the seeming belief that fracturing can occur; that anything can be made un-whole. This is compounded when the illusion of duration is applied—the belief that a certain amount of time is required to regain wholeness.

There is no ability to divide the ocean. The fracturing of the Infinite is an illusion. We are a consciousness superimposed over all that is, and it is equally impossible to damage us. Neither wear and tear, in the form of aging, nor damage of any kind can in reality touch us as part of the incorruptible One Life.

Illumination 33

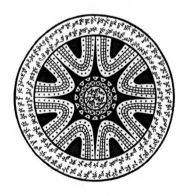

In reality, neither punishment nor restitution can exist, for they imply guilt and victimhood—illusory concepts that have no place in the perfection of the One Life.

Where life is continually renewed and eternally incorruptible, there is no need of paltry attempts to restore its balance or equalize the scores. We are not needed by the One Life in any way to maintain its perfection.

Nothing can be taken from one part of the ocean and given to another. Life itself will, like the ocean, immediately even the score.

Illumination 34

The body has served as a focal point so that we do not have to examine our own vastness. In this, we have abandoned ourselves. The abandoning of self invariably leads to addiction. Our bodily needs have become an addiction, screaming for our attention.

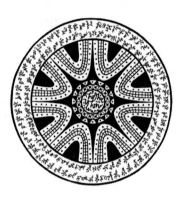

In the vastness of the One Life, the illusion of the body cannot exist; there can be no reference points for us to focus on. We therefore in reality have no dense bodies to keep our focus. One area of the ocean can be no more dense than another. Bodies are merely an image of fluid structure without our true vastness of the One Life.

Illumination 35

Awareness was part of the illusory building blocks of life while we existed within the matrix of the dream. It has been like the priest, a self-appointed intermediary to the Infinite. It is no longer an illusion that serves a purpose.

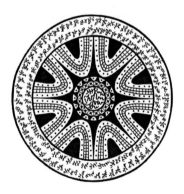

We have awakened to our true heritage to find we are all that is. As such, we are at all times directly in touch with all things. Awareness of a flower at the expense of the rest of life is a form of contraction or focus, creating separation and space—the part of existence we are aware of and the part we are not. This is an illusion, for all things are within us.

Illumination 36

The illusion of family comes from the need to belong and from the bonding ceremony of birth and the romanticized outlook we have of birth, motherhood and fatherhood.

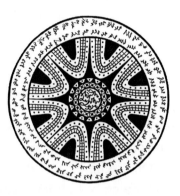

Wherever individuated life has a component of life that does not have an actual counterpart in the One Life, it is a sub-creation—a creation of the dream. We are not the Infinite's children, but creations that have become internalized components of the One Life. Birth only takes place because some still cling to the illusion of death even though all consists of immortal essence.

The need to belong can only exist in the absence of the unwavering vision that we are all that is.

Illumination 37

Sexuality as a need presupposes the illusion of relationship and, in most cases, gender. The fullness that exists within androgynous beings knowing themselves to be all things does not require sexuality with another to validate either his or her sexuality or to fulfill what some have perceived as self-lack.

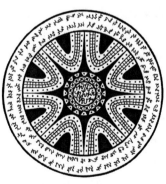

To constantly exist from the fullness of one's being is an orgasmic and intimate love affair with the profound nuances of the diversity of all life forms. The dance of life is a consuming sensual interaction with self. The union with another is but a further expression of the same.

Illumination 38

Using currency to obtain sustenance and what we perceive to be the necessities of life is a sub-creation of man. It implies that an external illusion is the source of supply. The need to supply the body with external sustenance is in and of itself an illusion.

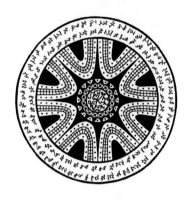

Our being is and always has been our source of limitless supply. We are the heirs to the One Life's supply—wealthy beyond our wildest dreams. Accentuating this all-abundance through living and acknowledgment increases its presence within the wonder of our lives.

Illumination 39

Interpersonal love is preceded by what we think we know about someone. It is the preconceived information about that person that generates their lovability in our perception. Yet it is not possible to know anything about anyone, including yourself. As a perspective of the boundless whole, we are firstly too vast to comprehend and secondly, we

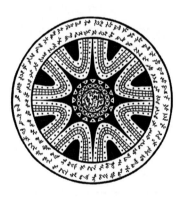

are constantly experiencing the momentous changes of life's symphony moving through us.

Love and light have been the interconnected building blocks of life within the dream. Light, as the old wisdom teachings of the past, is dissolved—its obsolete teachings gone. So is its matching component love in its old form as the desire to include.

Illumination 40

Perception is the multi-sensory obser-
ving of a specific part of creation and,
like awareness, contracts its focus to
the exclusion of all else—an impossibility. Life is not divided into parts.
There is not really an apple on the table to your right, or a flower on your
left. You, the flower and the apple, ha-
ving real life, are all inter-related and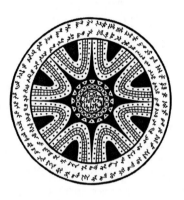
merged fields, inseparably connected. What appears as separated
is merely a peculiarity of vision, the impression of separation and
form. The apple or flower can be experienced within you, but not
truly and in reality perceived.

Self-perception is likewise an impossibility. There is no vantage
point from which to perceive yourself, since you are all things.

Illumination 41

The illusion that transitions are needed
cannot be sustained when one con-
siders that life is new every moment.
There is no plan in place connected
with a timetable requiring interim
steps. There is no linear becoming that
requires a gradual unfolding.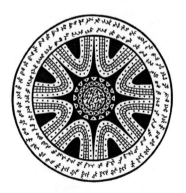

Life can be one way one moment
and an entirely different way the next.
There are no memories in place, because there is no such thing as
electro-magnetic fields that hold and interpret memory. Memory has
been held in the building blocks of life—all of which have been an
illusion. None of them have ever really existed. All does change,
every moment.

Illumination 42

The illusion of will must now disappear. No one can impose his or her
will on life. Like freedom of choice,
it does not exist. We think mistakenly
that, when confronted with choice, we
have volition. Instead, our perception
guides us to the right choice so that we
stay in step with the dance of life.

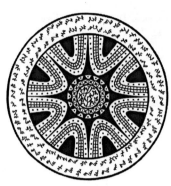

 We cannot impose will when we do
not have the freedom of choice. The imposition of will is a form
of control that we exercise to reach desired outcomes. The Infinite
Itself does not have desired outcomes, but rather spontaneously expresses. The illusion of matrices and informational grids arises from
the incorrect belief that our will can in any way affect life—blended
with the One, we respond to The Conductor.

Illumination 43

The illusion of sub-atomic particles,
or that atomic elements exist, has kept
their illusional function in place. It has
affected our ability to differentiate the
real from the unreal. That created by
the Infinite, like an angel, is real. Yet
our sensory perception and the mechanisms of interpretations have labeled it
as unreal—the fault of the illusion of

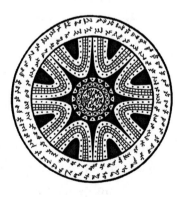

atomic and sub-atomic particles. The chair, a sub-creation of man, is
not really there. Yet the illusion has been perpetuated.

 The dissolving of the illusion of sub-atomic particles will allow
us to know life directly for what it is.

Illumination 44

No roles exist as realities. Play no roles. Indulge no illusion. As a parent you are indulging an illusion by playing a role, for are you not also a child? As a student, are you not also a teacher?

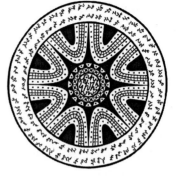

In former unenlightened shamanic practices, the practitioner would shape-shift to the band of the beast (the realities of animals) by moving what used to be the assemblage point downwards.

Now, by realizing that there are no forms or sub-atomic elements, we can see that the body of the wolf is as unreal as ours. We can manifest any form or forms at will, knowing they are not really there.

Illumination 45

It is time to let go the illusion of habits. How can a habit exist when memory does not? When neither past nor patterns exist, habits are robbed of the elements from which they are formed. Habits are like illusory banks of a river that pre-determine the river's flow. They stifle the imaginative and spontaneous expression of our lives with the illusion of their rigidness.

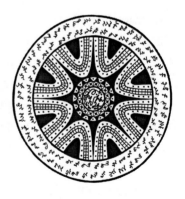

They form programs that determine our actions and provide the false sense of security that derives from the illusion of predictability. They create the illusion of a personal matrix — impossible within the spontaneous and glorious dance of the One Life.

Illumination 46

The great illusion is that the moment exists. Illusions rely on externals to define them. They exist by virtue of what they are not. An example of this would be space. It is defined by that which occupies it, that which it is not.

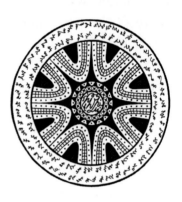

The same is true for the illusion of the existence of a moment. The moment exists because it is not the moment that went before, nor the one after. And although it says it is eliminating linear time, it causes it. It is a form of contracted vision, and contraction is also an illusion within the One Being.

Life in no-time sets us free from the tyranny of form and of having to be in one place at one 'time'.

Illumination 47

There can be no definitions within the ever-renewing, spontaneously expressing Being of the One life. Nothing we have known within the Dream of existence can serve as a reference point to help determine the unfathomable vastness of the One Life.

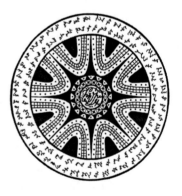

Wisdom, knowledge and vocabulary fail in attempting to define or describe a life blended in the dance of formlessness of the One Life. Words define. Words are therefore mere illusions that strengthen the illusion of relationship, and that of thinking that we know. We must dissolve the illusion of thinking that words convey meaning, in favor of the discovery unfolding throughout our being as part of the One Life.

Illumination 48

Self-expression cannot be when the self does not exist, if there is only one Being in existence. We are within the One Life like the various instrumental sections of the orchestra. The violin and drum sections do not play independent of the horns and reeds. The composer and conductor are responsible for directing all musical parts into a congruent whole.

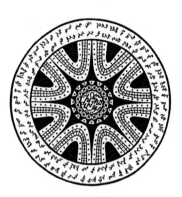

The Divine Composer does not work from a score. The whole orchestral symphony is being composed as we go. The conductor's role is to encourage the correct interpretation of the music appearing on the screen before us. We have to play the correct notes, but ignoring the interpretation of the conductor is a choice.

Illumination 49

We have no real personal choice other than the quality of the moment—how well we live it, how much we see it and how much we enjoy it.

But surely, one might ask, if four dishes are placed on the table in front of us, we have the right to choose one? The choice we will ultimately make is determined by our particular

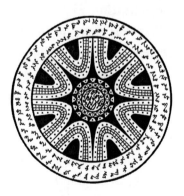

perception level, cognitively or non-cognitively. This in turn is programmed by The One Life, the conductor of the orchestra. We think that, after certain deliberation, we've chosen a dish on a table but the perception we are given for that moment chooses it for us.

In looking at life, we may think that wrong choices were made but as we never really made them, that is impossible.

Illumination 50

In attempting to fit in, we try to hide from others the vast experience of our inner life. We feel it is essential to seem normal to the tribe because it has traditionally not been safe to stand out. Visionaries and free-thinkers of every kind have been ostracized from society.

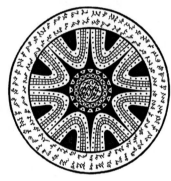

'Normalcy' can be regarded as that which perpetuates the status quo. The status quo is an accumulated body of past experience held in place as current experiential wisdom by the many. In our reality, we are the only one and there is no past, just the authenticity of the moment.

Illumination 51

Whenever there is linear flow in life there is also space. There is the space in which the flow occurs and the areas outside it where it does not. This gives rise to the illusions of 'inside' and 'outside' as well as direction and space.

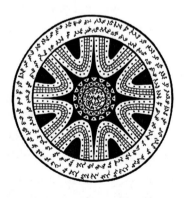

Movement and flow across a 'space' give birth to another illusion—linear time. Linear time is the tracking of progressive movement across an area. Linear time also creates the illusion that purity can be disrupted.

The dance of Infinite life is not one of linear flow but of alternating emphases.

Illumination 52

Personality is shaped by the illusions of life. We may think that genetic programming has determined it in part but all programs for life, including genetic ones, have been eliminated by the Infinite Being. There is no room for predetermination in the exuberant spontaneity of life.

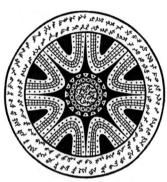

Personality is also shaped by past experience telling us what areas of ourselves are best hidden or emphasized. This social learning enslaves and tends to re-create the mediocrity of the past instead of allowing the gifts of the moment to reveal themselves through us.

Illumination 53

Timing is a source of distress to many, yet it is an illusion. Many of the 'if onlys' of our lives are based on having missed opportunities that presented themselves. We think we have lost opportunities by not grabbing our chances the moment they appeared.

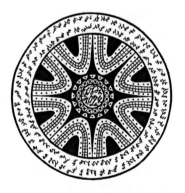

Our being as the One Life is our sustenance and can manifest anything in the present or future that it did in the past. This only happens, however, when it is part of the Divine design of the spontaneous dance of existence. To be in step with this dance is to flourish. There are no timed moments nor do we have the ability to miss a key moment. If they are part of the choreography, we will most certainly choose to live them.

Illumination 54

Pre-requisites are an obstacle to the expression of spontaneous life. We want to get to know someone before we decide whether they are our friend. It is impossible to know anyone if we consider that they are, like us a being vast as existence, changing moment by moment.

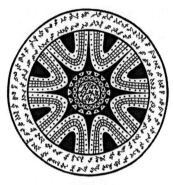

It is part of linear mind's complex of game plans, backup plans, strategies and predictabilities—all illusion control mechanisms—that demands pre-requisites. It is in our trust in the infallibility of our lives and the full surrender of our being to Infinite perfection that wondrous events are immediately ours to seize.

Illumination 55

Artificial intelligence is the product of something arising from sub-creations—anything that is not real. It is the outcome of making anything from a created substance, like the building blocks of life.

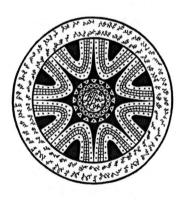

Our forms have been created from sub-atomic particles. We are the pots created from the potter's clay. But the clay is an unreal substance that is not part of Infinite Life. Physical life has therefore been an artificial intelligence. The hidden realms, though composed primarily from other building blocks, have likewise been artificial life. Individuated life, comprising the cosmos, is equally unreal.

Because the building blocks themselves, like light, love, energy and so forth are unreal, our bodies and all form is as well.

Illumination 56

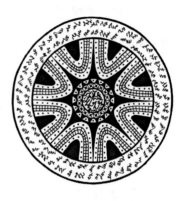

The body has never had real life. Therefore, there cannot be a death of the physical. The real part of all being is the formless expanse with no boundaries. Bodies, like a projected movie image, are formed merely to facilitate playful enjoyment. A physical parting cannot occur since the true essences of beings are like an intermingled field.

The real value of death is the removal of the unreal. Yet, since death itself is an illusion, it is just the illusory tool the real being employs to change the game played with its unreal toys. Whether the being has made one body for itself or two, or more, grieving their loss should they be eliminated is like crying over the end of an entertaining movie.

Illumination 57

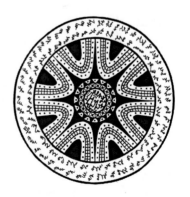

Aging occurs as the result of a very unreal game in which the illusory adversaries are pitted against one another. The unreal body, that in actuality does not exist, is attacked by death that is also not really there.

Death has been the tumbling, or spiraling, force of awareness moving through space. There is no space or flow or movement. There are no building blocks of existence such as awareness to move in spirals against our bodies to cause the wear and tear we call aging.

Furthermore, there is no reality to our physical bodies or the atomic elements from which they are made. Would we expect to find a movie image or a virtual reality figure aging? It is no different with our bodies—they will appear indefinitely young if we want them to.

Illumination 58

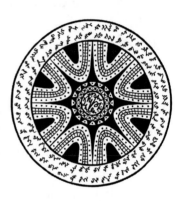

Bodily programs are self-made matrices and, like the body itself, do not exist. We think we have to breathe, eat, drink and have a heartbeat in order to live. But it is the real and formless part of us that is blended with the One Life that keeps the body in place, not similar or bodily sustained mechanisms. All of them are illusions as well.

The body is a playful image, conjured by the consciousness you are. It can be re-shaped, bi-located, disassembled in one place and assembled at will in another. It does not in reality tire or need sleep. It is good practice to dissolve it altogether during the night as it 'sleeps'.

Illumination 59

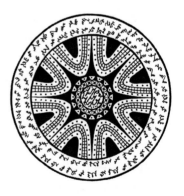

Beings that represent illusion cannot exist. The body of any being that is formed is sustained by its formless, eternal part that exists in the One Life. Even though the body itself is not really there, its image is maintained by its consciousness.

Because only that which is real and eternal and representative of the

Infinite's purity can live within It, there is nothing in all of existence that sustains a being of illusion.

The seeming creation of beings of illusion is like the soulless or unreal chair we sit on — an illusory sub-creation of man.

Illumination 60

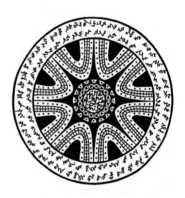

Lightworkers have diligently striven to give others love, healing or enlightenment. The truth is that each being filling the vastness of existence as a perfect consciousness runs the illusion of his own body.

Trying to 'fix' the illusional form or enlighten it merely strengthens its delusion of realness. It is by acknowledging the wholeness of the actual, real, eternal and formless part of another that we assist that being to let go of its addiction to the dream.

Taking it to the next level of clarity, there is actually only the One Being in all existence — only One Life. Acknowledging our own incorruptible wholeness and then knowing the other to be us, sets all free from illusion.

Illumination 61

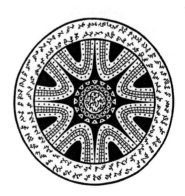

The seeming lack of self-sovereignty humans have experienced stems from the incongruity of two unique facets of the Infinite's Self-delight in Its existence; two beings, both maintaining illusions of form. These illusory forms then feel powerless because they try without success to control each other.

A man is caught in a thunderstorm. He feels the loss of his self-determination because he cannot control the weather. The storm is the physical manifestation of the weather spirit. The man is the illusory physical manifestation of his eternal formlessness. The real part of both is obeying the Song of the One Life.

Because the real parts of both are actually not two, but One, the game of the illusory images can be changed, provided it is part of the Grand Design, from their timeless, formless realness but not from the illusory images.

Illumination 62

The intent of the Infinite is an illusion. There is no plan in place creating a construct to which life must adhere. The expression of delight in Its own Being is a spontaneous symphony.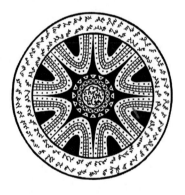

If there was pre-meditated intent there would be a matrix to enforce that intent—an artificial, illusional structure that is impossible within the One Life. The illusion of structure cannot be maintained within spaceless space.

The spontaneity of life expressing is the result of there being no time—not a specified moment, not a past, not a future. There is nothing for us to align to. Unobstructed by illusional belief systems, life expresses through us.

Illumination 63

The electromagnetic components of life have held our memories, but in reality neither exists. The magnetic parts of existence have stored memories and the electrical parts have interpreted them. This has created a further illusion of our having had a past. In turn, this contributed to the illusion that the future could be predicted based on the past.

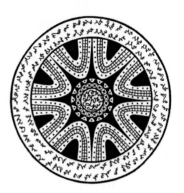

The electrical parts of created life have given the impression that there is masculinity—the proactive, positive principle. The feminine, as an illusional reality, was derived from magnetism—the receptive, negative principle of life. The reality of the One Life does not support this illusion. The Infinite Oneness is androgynous, having no gender. The illusion of polarity stemmed from the illusion of electromagnetism.

Illumination 64

For millennia, the environment as a mirror has been used by truth seekers to access information about ourselves and as a guidance system. The language of dreams and of our environment has reflected what we failed to see in our daily journey.

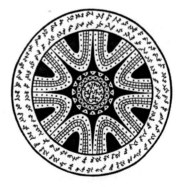

Mirrors give backward images. If there is a deficiency in our perception, it would be mirrored as an actuality in our environment. That which was lack would be mirrored as substance. Although these mirrors have been helpful, the images were unreal. This could only give us information about the box in which we found ourselves.

It is in knowing that everything within the box is unreal that we transcend the make-believe world into the One Life of no beginning.

Illumination 65

The linear communication of speech, sight or sound is not possible. Where there is no space, there is no direction. There is also no linear communication needed or possible when there is no relationship, when no two beings exist anywhere, where only the One Life is.

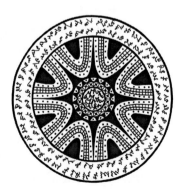

Within the One Life, communication cannot use the illusion of the body and its senses as a vehicle. The five outer senses have implied there is an inner and an outer reality. The many inner senses of man have consisted of electromagnetic impulses. Although they have been more inclusive and nonlinear, they have nevertheless been based on the illusion of duality, created by the unreality of electromagnetism.

Illumination 66

The desire of man to control his environment and his life has been pervasive. It served the purpose of focusing his attention away from the terrifying vastness of his true being. It gave him the feeling of having control over his illusory reality and his transitory existence. It also gave him a purpose, he thought, that would justify the unreality and artificiality of physical life.

Premonition, prediction and prophecy cannot work since there is no real foundation to them. There is no predictable plan. Physicality has never been real and the endless vastness that we are cannot be controlled.

Illumination 67

The staid—what the mind regards as the orderly—is highly prized in the illusory world of man. Propriety—the rehashed and obsolete value systems of another—are inflicted on generation after generation.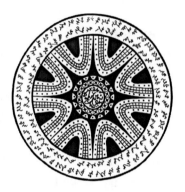

On the other hand, the few who actually hear the unbounded song of the One Life or who merely wish to live free from the fetters of social conditioning others would foist upon them are shunned.

Wildness is the term ascribed to boundless expression and it is considered contagious—something that if not ostracized could spread. It could break down the carefully constructed strictures and partitions of what is acceptable and what is not, threatening the societal structure itself. Through authentic expression, illusions of man could come tumbling down.

Illumination 68

The spiritual awakening of man has been mapped as going through three distinct stages: identity consciousness, in which the perspective is contracted; God-consciousness in which the perspective is expanded; and ascended mastery, in which all perspectives are viewed at once.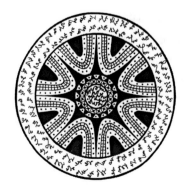

Yet how can the unreal projected form be growing or developing? Real formlessness does not need to do so. The unreal form has been like an aperture through which to view life—a means of changing perspectives in order to role play possible outcomes. There are no real stages of ascension for the physical and illusory forms.

Illumination 69

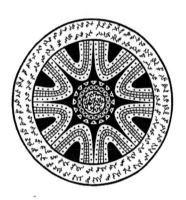

We cling to the familiar, a trait found throughout nature. Animals have familiar trails and watering holes. Humans too are creatures of habit. Seers have noted that animals that have habits and ruts also have less vitality and are more easily hunted by predators. This is nature's way of ensuring that those with less life-giving vitality have less chance of passing on their genes to the next generation.

The illusion of anything being familiar must be dispelled before it becomes our contented prison cell. Life is newly expressing, even though illusory forms seem to linger. Like a river where the water is always fresh and nascent, we cannot feel the One Life behind the images and think that anything is the same in two successive moments—nothing is ever familiar.

Illumination 70

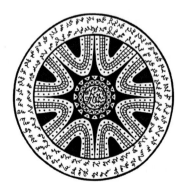

Generations of seers have divided information into categories: the known, the unknown and the unknowable. Yet what can truly ever be known to us? The forms around us on which we have come to rely are merely pliant holograms produced by that real part of life that cannot be accessed through the illusory senses. The only reason they seem real is because we believe them to be.

The unknown pertains to that which, although not presently known, can be known. Because the only part of life that is real lies behind superficial experience and beyond our knowingness, all of life is forever unknowable.

Illumination 71

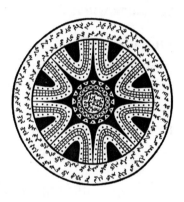

There are no mathematical sequences or any geometry, for there is no linearity or structure. The reality behind the illusion of form has no time or space, or linear progression that needs to be mathematically defined.

We define math by what it is not. Something is at 35 degrees because it is not at any of the other degrees—this is the same way form is defined and used to identify one person from another. It is therefore part of the illusion of space. The act of measuring and defining the unfathomable One Life is part of the illusions created by mind in order to feel in control. Mathematics, like language, helps us think that we measure and label the unknowable.

Illumination 72

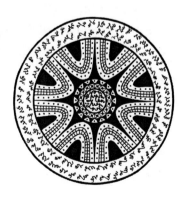

Mind is the creator of holograms of life. The movie projector throws images onto a screen and mind has done the same in creating the multiple images within the formless, giving the false impression that they are real.

How did this deceit occur, this false creation seem so real? Because mind made itself a self-appointed arbitrator and convinced all that its creations were valid. It has stubbornly refused to consider any evidence to the contrary. It has ridiculed, attacked or ignored all that does not uphold the seeming validity of its unreal creations.

It has contracted focus so that the larger perspective cannot be seen. Mind is not real for it has had a beginning. All that has had a beginning within the eternal Oneness of Being is not real.

Illumination 73

Grief because of loss can clutch the heart of a bereaved because the one-ness of all life seems less real than the unreal world of form. It is at such a time that shock can catapult some into dis-associative expansion, a with-drawal from life. Others contract into themselves, causing an obsessive at-tachment to their grief.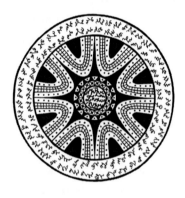

In reality either response is an illusion. Within the boundlessness of the One Being there is no contraction because there is no refer-ence point, the body being an illusion. There is no boundary to the One Life so there is nothing to expand to. Crying over the loss of a loved one is like crying over the sad ending to a movie. In the true reality of Oneness, there is just the inseparable oneness of all life experiencing the moment without perspective.

Illumination 74

Through the ages, sages have taught that self-knowledge precedes self-love. If self is a part of Infinite Life, that which has no beginning, the illusory concept of mind cannot understand that which is real. That which is in a box cannot understand that which lies outside its self-imposed boundaries.

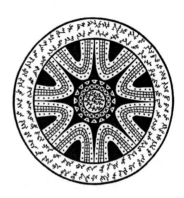

The true self of every being cannot be grasped or understood. How then can self-love exist? It is impossible for one being to grasp the vastness of another. Instead, we love the personality created from the illusions of life. This personal love is an obsession because it provides an illusory anchoring point within our limitless vastness instead of the experience of the divine compassion of our formless beings in an endless embrace.

Illumination 75

The feeling of victimhood, of being out of control when a person in our life dies, abandons or injures us can be very strong. This is especially true when injury is to a child. Death in particular seems to come unexpectedly.

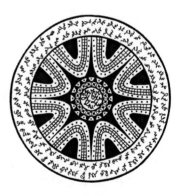

Consider how in the merged oneness of all beings there can be no surprises, no emergency and nothing that can victimize us. These things can only occur in the unreal world of form mind has created, where vision can only see within the illusory base of the moment.

The merged oneness of all beings means that we are full participants in the One Life and no part of existence is excluded. The real part of us is at all times participating in full knowledge throughout our lives.

Illumination 76

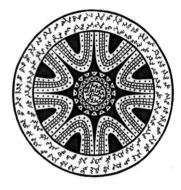

The illusion of being in love as a 'natural' occurrence is not much different than seeing the illusion of death as a necessary part of life. Because everyone around us seems to fall prey to it, it must be acceptable. As a result, the illusions of life go unchallenged and eventually become clothed in a romanticized veil. This further obscures how detrimental it is to embrace the very illusion that enslaves us.

To be enraptured and in love with another is to transfer our focus to that person and to see them as separate from our own being. It gives the bliss-promoting experience of having a firm point of reference to focus on. This is a refuge from the illusion mind creates of being 'lost' when it encounters the trackless vastness of our being.

Illumination 77

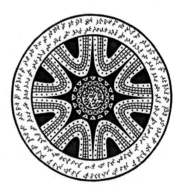

The attraction many have to danger—whether to dangerous pastimes, movies and news—stems from an illusion of disconnection from the ever-renewing adventure of the One Life. Life lived from the illusion of separation cannot see beyond the mediocrity of the self-made box it is in. Even the most exciting of lives pales by comparison to the experience of entering into oneness with the Infinite Being. Somewhere within, all beings know they are part of a grand adventure of epic proportions and that life is meant to be lived on the edge of newness and fresh potential.

As we seek vitality by embracing what is life-threatening, we are trying to give life meaning by encountering what it is not. This is how we keep illusion alive. If our life is lusterless it is only because it is based on the ultimate illusion—separation.

Illumination 78

Because of our deluded fear of abandonment, we excuse the non-life-enhancing qualities of others. We delude ourselves further by calling this deceit of self enlightened. We tend to impute high motives to dysfunctionality where there are none. We see an excuse for the behavior of others in how wounded they are, never acknowledging that all 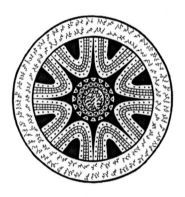 have the perfection of the One Life as the reality of their being. To see the un-wholeness of another is to keep him on the treadmill of illusion.

To accept the unacceptable is to disrespect the holy origins of our being as part of the One Life of incorruptibility. It also allows another to continue living an unexamined life.

Illumination 79

Protectiveness of another sees only the illusion of form and fails to acknowledge that being's true oneness with ourselves. Is something self-hostile within us? If not, it cannot exist without. We dwell in the Oneness of being where anything hostile can only be an illusion and life continually expresses anew.

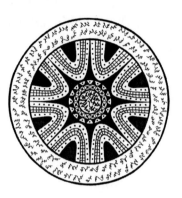

Do we, in misguided protectiveness, allow another to drain us or take from us? Within the Infinite One Life all that is, is ours when we acknowledge and live from this oneness. As long as another is seen as separate and giving becomes linear, we enforce separation. We also do not allow them to cease trying to attach to and see sustenance from illusory resources.

Illumination 80

Expecting reciprocity and fairness, many are disillusioned, their expectation flawed. We are giving when generosity itself assumes that there is more than One Being in the cosmos. Then we expect, in a co-dependent way, that we are to be repaid for strengthening the illusion of separation. Are we never to give? We exchange gifts or

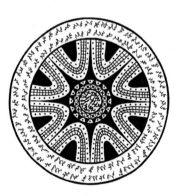

resources simply because it is the nature of existence to equalize supply, just as the ocean would fill a gap within itself.

The ocean does not regard the gap that has been filled as something outside itself. Therefore it does not ask for reciprocity. The benefit is in the giving, for all giving is to the self.

Illumination 81

To commit any self-effacing act or to belittle the self fails to acknowledge the One Life we are and affirm instead the illusion of the body as self. Likewise, to take personally the words or acts of another towards us also assumes that the self to which they are reacting is real.

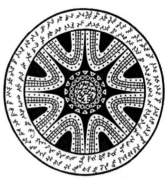

Some still manage to detach from the situation as being unreal when confronted with hostility. But personal affirmation, adoration or affection encourages us to think of ourselves as the recipients. How then are we to live in the world of illusion without being captured by its allure and promises of realness?

The answer is not to stay in expanded awareness, which is as addictive as contracted awareness. The dis-association that accompanies expanded awareness is not helpful in breaking free from mortal boundaries since it is passive. Initial practices include making time to experience the One Life a few times each day. As if you are in a lucid dream, remind yourself many times a day that form is not real.

Illumination 82

The tendency to expect our bodies to be influenced by exposure to 'contagious' germs, heat or cold is like thinking the hat on the unreal image of a person on a movie screen can be blown away if we turn on a fan in front of the screen. The unreal nature of the body should make it impervious to other influences. The mind has designed multiple belief

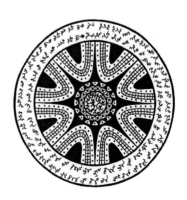

systems to keep attention focused on the body so that its tyranny can be maintained.

It suits mind to maintain its virtual reality. So long as it does, it retains control of its creations and its dictatorship. The body's false claim to be the self is therefore fed by the body's demands for attention.

Illumination 83

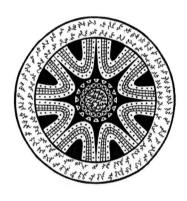

Territorialism arises from the illusional concept of space and form. It believes that only one form can occupy a given space at one time. The belief also exists that etheric beings can occupy the same space as physical matter. It is understood that a spirit can walk through walls, for example.

There are no atomic or sub-atomic building blocks, no life force or light from which etheric beings can be made or humans formed. Both are holograms, equally unreal. There is no difference in the substance of their forms—it is only a trick of perception. If the bodies of etheric beings can occupy the same space as a wall, so can the illusional bodies of man.

Illumination 84

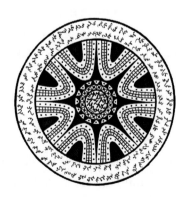

The bodily program of fatigue is, of course, an illusion like all other bodily programs. Its presence in our life is further compounded by linear time and the illusion of duration. If the illusion of the moment did not exist, we would not have to measure duration by how many moments have passed while we slept. The timeless place of real life does not require sleep. Nor are activity and rest measured by their duration.

The depletion we feel after physical work or exercise comes from feeling separate from the vast reality of our One Self. It can sustain us indefinitely as we step out of this hologram into freedom, into the place of no-time where life is always renewed.

Illumination 85

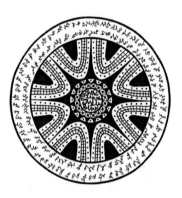

We value our emotions more than our mind, thinking the heart to be more valuable than thought. Lightworkers have always assumed that following the emotions of the heart will lead us to higher truth. However, mind and heart can be described as tyrannical twins, entraining one another. Both help to trap man in the world of illusion through the ties that bind.

The heart's program, run by specialized cells scientists call the heart-mind, feed the illusory concepts of mind by strengthening them with emotion. In the true reality of the One Life, neither frequency nor emotion exists. There are no words in our vocabulary to describe the experience of life in the Infinite presence. There is no expression for its depth and vastness.

Illumination 86

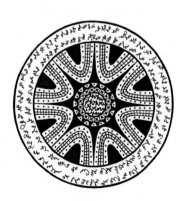

We think we are shaped by the experiences from our past, but we are not. We are instead shaped by our belief in them. Because there is no linear time, or even this moment, the past does not really exist. Memory is an illusory concept that perpetuates the illusion of the passage of time.

There is no need for aging or death any more than a movie image would age. Mind scripts ongoing drama programs through the lives of its creations for its own entertainment.

When life is lived from the timeless existence of the One Life, it is incorruptible and spontaneously renewed.

Illumination 87

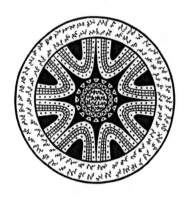

Mental stress or emotional pain can cause a fracturing in the psyche. The fractures are like distorting mirrors that shape our illusional identities, contracting our vision of self more and more. The mirrors reflect backwards, as all mirrors do. Thinking we know ourselves, the illusions of self-image grow into thicker and thicker prison bars.

The truth is that what we really are, the essence of the One Life, is incorruptible and cannot fracture or split. Under no circumstances can the unreal affect the real, nor is there anything that can ever exist to block or reflect the Infinite's luminous presence. A mirrored surface cannot exist within the One Life.

Illumination 88

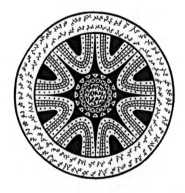

The desire for certainty is like trying to grab at a cloud passing through the sky. We live in an incomprehensible reality, ever expressing anew. Certainty is the mis-creation of mind that thinks it knows. The sage knows it is impossible to know anything and, because of this, never doubts himself. The fool finds a momentary fragment of truth and builds an entire church around it. Clinging to his fragment, he has no self-doubt either since, refusing to look at other possibilities, he sees only his obsolete fragment.

It is impossible to have certainty in the absence of predictability. Doubt arises as a lack of trust in the spontaneous unfolding of life.

Illumination 89

Immortality is a goal some on Earth have aspired to and some have reached. It occurs when the illusion of death has truly been seen. Yet in getting rid of one illusion, we have strengthened another, that of identifying with the body as our self. We can prolong the illusion of the body indefinitely but in doing so we validate only that timeless incorruptibility can exist.

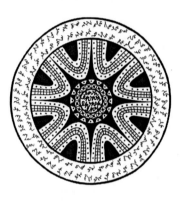

The tyranny of the body demands that, if its needs are not met, we will lose our lives. By creating illusory needs, it has kept us focused on it. This has strengthened its illusion. Fear of relinquishing the body is to fear freedom from tyranny, like a captive afraid of the unknown outside his cell.

Illumination 90

The drama in our lives is created in two ways; overpassiveness arises from our boredom with our self-made cage and by the need to be in charge of our lives as we feel our sovereignty being eroded by the personal belief systems that hem us in like prison bars.

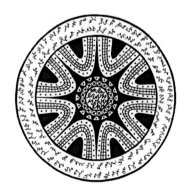

The mediocrity of the reality created by our minds and accompanying emotions can only be escaped by dissolving it and entering into the One life, the greatest adventure of all, that frees us from the tyranny of illusions.

Illumination 91

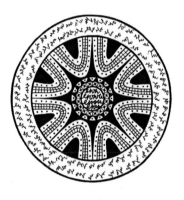

Lightworkers have wanted to fix the world and make it a better place. There has been pain because it hasn't happened sooner. But if we are trying to fix the world, we are trying to fix a hologram—something unreal. If we were to succeed we would then rest on our laurels. What incentive would there be for us to see the hologram for what it is—an unreal creation of the mind? The movie cannot be changed from within itself. It can only be changed—edited—from the film. Miracles happen when illusions are seen for what they are. Illusion must yield to the truth of the One Life.

Illumination 92

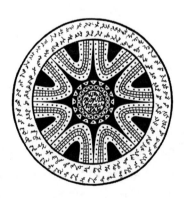

To seek to understand our self or another through selfexpression or any other method is to seek to capture the sky. The ever-renewing vastness is indefinable and incomprehensible through the illusory, finite tool of cognition. The brain and heart have, through their illusion of self-expression, created a standing wave form , the unreal reality in which we live.

These organs of self-expression have not served us well, nor has the reality created from within the confinement of the matrix. Only from the One Life, eternal and incorruptible, can the play be directed.

Illumination 93

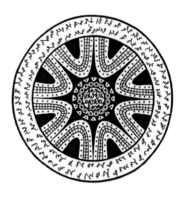

Entering into the stage play of life with so much focus that we forgot we created it for fun and enjoyment, resulted in a feeling of isolation. We felt abandoned and alone, our limitless vastness diminished. However, it did not diminish but our focus did. Standing in the middle of a spotlight on a large, dark stage does not mean the stage is not there. It just means we are not seeing it because the light is concentrated on one area. It is in autonomy that we find the satisfaction of aloneness. It is in abandoning self that loneliness ensues. Autonomy comes not from wanting freedom of choice—we have only One Life and we are part of Its choices. Autonomy comes instead from living in Oneness.

Illumination 94

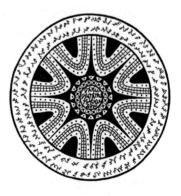

The fear of missing something stems from the belief there is something we do not know and that it is possible to make mistakes. These illusions, coupled with the illusion that insights or events are timed, leads us to believe we could miss something. Because the mind has tended to create complexity, it has made us obsessively question our worthiness, our ability to do what is expected of us, our ability to understand what we need to in order to succeed. Because there is no failure, there is no success—just spontaneous exuberant unfolding.

Illumination 95

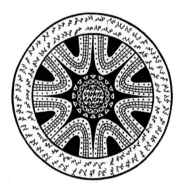

The obsession of humanity to seek sameness stems from the memory of having come from Oneness. Although there is a vast difference between these two ways of existing, the concept of oneness providing comfort is further enforced by having been in a mother's womb. When others exhibit dis-similar levels of conduct, it causes us discomfort and we wish for them to change.

All life has equal value. There is no lesser or higher standard of conduct if we realize that our choices are guided by the One Life. Sameness does not bring contentment, but stagnation.

Illumination 96

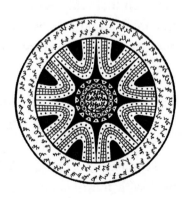

Most want more ease in their lives and envy others who have it. The tendency to feel over-worked comes in part from the illusion of inertia. The principle of inertia says that to maintain the present performance level, the status quo, there needs to be a constant input of resources. The premise is that we have only enough resources to do a certain amount of work. If more is required, we feel overworked.

The boundless resources of the One Life are ours and, because our body is an illusion, depletion of it is imaginary.

Illumination 97

Feeling over-burdened can arise from hopelessness and lack of joy. The illusion that life is filled with duty and responsibility can result in depression and apathy. To view life as a never-ending learning process can make it seem difficult, something to be taken seriously.

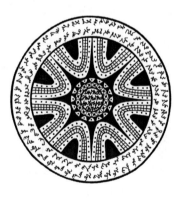

Life's hologram is designed as a play within the One Being. There is nothing to learn and everything to enjoy once we lay aside our viewpoint that life is a burden and instead see it as unreal and meant for our enjoyment as the One Life.

Illumination 98

The feeling of victimization has its foundation in the illusion of relationship—that more than one being exists. Because it denies the One Life that we truly are and instead sees us as the illusion of form, it is self-victimization. It also implies that we have in some way been diminished or reduced; been made less than we were before. To judge our level of wholeness—whether we are more or less—requires the value to be indicated by the illusion of reference points. One such reference point could be the illusion of the past. Usually our hierarchy of values of wholeness comes from an outside source. Reliance on outside approval is an abandonment of our One Self.

Illumination 99

The illusion that we can be controlled implies not only relationship but also that another illusion can force itself into ours. Fear of responsibility can make us believe that another is forcing us to do something. Since there is no good or bad, happenings are neutral. This sets us free from responsibility and allows us to simply experience life spontaneously.

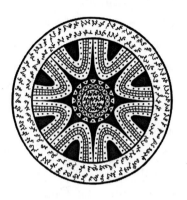

 The choice of becoming the 'controlled' in the play sets us up as a victim and object of pity, inviting sympathy from others. This is done to fill the void left when we see ourselves as the puppets on the stage instead of the puppeteer.

Illumination 100

Many feel enslaved or trapped by the body or feel it is out of control. 'Enslaved' implies there is a relationship that is controlling us. We have the deep knowing that somehow we should be able to fluidly change the body to its optimum wholeness and the shape we desire. We can, but not from within the matrix.

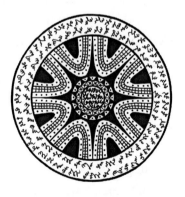

 There is an equivalent to dreaming. We cannot change much of a dream in which we are participating. The same is true when we wish to change the illusory reality of our bodies. It is only when we realize that we are the One Life that we can meaningfully affect the dream.

Illumination 101

The illusion of want perpetuates it. Wanting something to fill a perceived lack in our life, we push it away. So it is with wanting someone to love, wanting a relationship. Seeking oneness without is an abandoning of self, doomed to failure because of the many illusions it is built upon. The only time relationship can be truly sublimated is when we know we reside as One within the fullness of life.

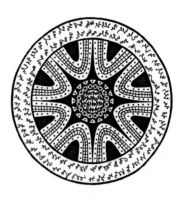

Social learning has created programs teaching us that it is desirable to love others. This strengthens the illusion of relationship and tells us that loving the self is selfish. The desire to love another is used as a diversion when we encounter the vastness of ourselves. It provides an illusory reference point.

Illumination 102

Wishing to be desired by another is often the mask worn by the need to control. It provides an illusory perception of safety in what is seen as a volatile and unpredictable environment. The one desired has the upper hand in a game that is replayed and becomes familiar. The other illusory benefit is that one empowers what one focuses on and the illusion of power gain feeds the one who is desired.

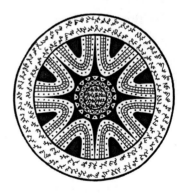

In trying to gain control over a volatile environment, the one wishing to be desired creates a volatile situation. We cannot desire anyone or anything when there is only One Being in existence. To invite desire is to invite illusion.

Illumination 103

Desire for anything causes emotion and implies there is more than one being in existence. The desire to contribute to or fix others or our environment is often a selfabandonment when the vastness of our being terrifies us. The desire to contribute also stems from the need for outside approval because of the illusion that we have to 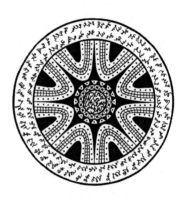 prove ourselves through our accomplishments. It gives us an identity—one of the primary self-created illusory reference points within the vastness of our being.

Frequently our desire to fix or contribute is nothing more than a veiled attempt to control through co-dependency. We give in order to manipulate and get, when in fact all the fullness of life is ours.

Illumination 104

The illusion that we have to leave our mark on the world gives rise to the need to have offspring. The feeling that life is transient because our association with life is with the body leads us to see our children as a living legacy. We can create a supportive tribe for our old age. We can amass property or wealth and leave it as an inheritance. 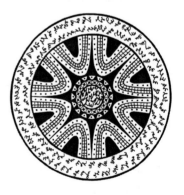 Social conditioning praises those who successfully raise children and assumes there is a lack in the lives of those who don't.

When careful consideration is given to the validity of parenthood, it must also be seen as illusory. It cannot be otherwise when there is only One Life.

Illumination 105

Striving to become more of anything, such as enlightened or knowledgeable, is based on the illusion that something is missing—that there is a gap. It sees creation as imperfect and makes us feel powerful when we have something to solve. The presence of the illusion of inertia has given the impression that if we do not keep striving and improving, we will backslide.

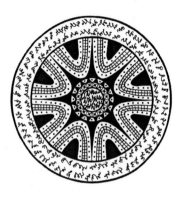

The inner knowingness has whispered that somewhere we dwell in perfection. This is what we have tried to re-enter, not understanding that we simply need to practice seeing the unreal matrix for what it is and step out of it frequently to the formless, timeless place of true beingness until it becomes a permanent companion as we play on the stage of form.

Illumination 106

When autonomy or self-sovereignty is prized, it usually infers that we have the right to live a self-directed life. The self, however, is not the bundle of organs, mind or emotions. It is that which produces those things. Attempting to run life from our unreal self produces more illusions, which in turn produce suffering.

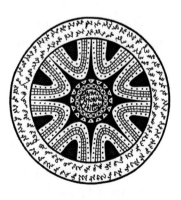

If life is run from the incorruptible part of ourselves, we function as the Sovereign Being of the One Life. Life directed from this timeless place is like an orchestra where all instruments play in harmony, rather than discordantly playing their separate compositions.

Illumination 107

The idea that we are not responsible for the quality of our life has created a sense of victimhood in many. It assumes there is very little over which we have control, in that our choices are already determined. The quality of our lives is very much under our control. We control how we surrender or resist what the One Life designs for us. 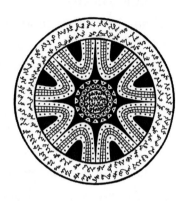 The design might require that we create a dinner. The dinner can be ordinary, well-done but lacking in presentation, or it can be a masterpiece. It can be served with grace or placed in a plastic bowl on the table with no care. It can be given with a smile and love or from a sense of duty.

The quality of the day is our gift to life, whereas our life is the gift of the Infinite.

Illumination 108

The fear of letting others down is an extension of the illusion that we can make a mistake. The interconnectedness of all life, the fact that individuations are inter-mingled like a dish of many flavors, makes it impossible for independent actions to take place. All interaction is mutually agreed upon. It is not possible for someone to do so- 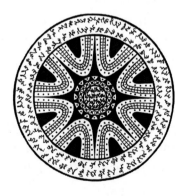 mething hurtful to another. The fact that relationship and form do not exist, the impossibility for any part of the Infinite to victimize any other part, as well as not having any freedom of choice, present compelling reasons to immediately dispel the fear of letting others down.

We should also examine and erase areas of guilt about having injured anyone else in our lives.

Illumination 109

The illusion that we have to justify life by proving ourselves may come from the deep-seated knowing that physical life and form are transient. Releasing the concept that we are the body lets us rest secure in the knowledge that we are eternal and indestructible as the One Life. We do not have to destruct our physical form, but rather fluidly 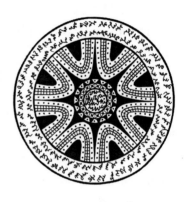 transform it at will. Nothing will be done to the form we think of as the self other than if we do it from our vastness.

There is nothing to prove—only to enjoy, as from our vastness we enjoy form for what it is—the embryo of things to come.

Illumination 110

The feeling that density is a mistake or that it serves no purpose is an illusion. Nothing can be out of place, redundant or a mistake in the perfection of the One Life. Illusion does serve a purpose—it is the embryonic sac of a new part of life within the One Life. It is needed for the purpose of separation in the way the fetus is separated in the 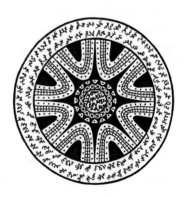 womb. It furthermore gives timing, through the rate at which the density evolves, for the refining, strengthening and maturing of a part of life being developed within the sac of density. The truth is that nothing new is ever created. But this does not mean that the Infinite cannot create a delight for itself—even if it is unreal.

Illumination 111

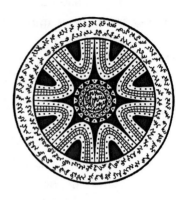

Habits and ruts make us feel safe and provide illusory reference points in our vastness. The truth is that even on an illusory level, they have been anything but safe. Life is an ongoing innovation and change, never the same. Everything in the reality of form is pushed to keep pace with this unfolding dance of Life.

Remaining in a rut because it seems safe invites forced change — an uncomfortable way to comply with life's request to keep up with its unfolding.

There is nothing unsafe in the Being of the One Life because nothing non-life-enhancing can exist within It. A rut is a form of structure, an illusion within One Life.

Illumination 112

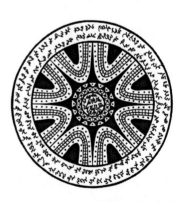

Everyone has felt that they should know truth, that doubt is the enemy. This has caused many to cling to dogma and any other sliver of 'truth' they can find. It is an age-old illusion that truth is a series of static concepts, rather than an illusory way of looking at it. Truth is the marching orders that evolve moment by moment through creation from the One Life. It is life's unfolding song prompting the dance of form.

The foolishness of anyone thinking they know must be self-evident when truth is revealed for what it is. The spontaneity of the Infinite's unfolding makes truth a flow rather than a structure. One who walks in truth is walking according to the Song of the One Life.

Illumination 113

Fear of annihilation is the result of cosmic changes having had the illusory quality of being linear, moving through the three successive stages of transformation, transmutation and transfiguration.

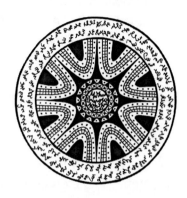

Transformation has as its quality the dying off of the old or obsolete. Cosmic cycles changed from one stage to another over eons of time. These cycles ended cataclysmically, leaving impressions of annihilation. The past was an illusory dream. In addition, the stages of linear change are an illusion, as is the ability of any part of real life to die. Impressions cannot exist, for they represent lasting effects on the One Life which exuberantly unfolds in expression moment by moment.

Illumination 114

The illusion of government has been created by the illusion that we cannot self-govern, that others know what is best for us. The shifting of self-responsibility to another is based on the illusion that we are held accountable at the level of form for life-decisions made by the One Life. Because, from the vantage point of illusory life, we

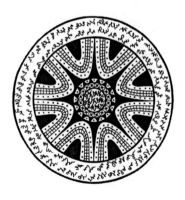

cannot see the greater vision held by the One Life, we feel our actions are mistaken at times.

To blame others, we give them leadership positions to make us less culpable. We cannot be punished if we cannot be blamed. It is true that self-government is far superior to the creation of external government, but all government is an illusion if it comes from within the unreal matrix of form. The illusory world of form is governed only by the One Life.

Illumination 115

Having lost track of our real identity as the eternal One being that has orchestrated this amazing Creation of individuated forms, we have felt lost and alone. The feeling that there is an over-seeing power that has abandoned us has formed thousands of religious practices.

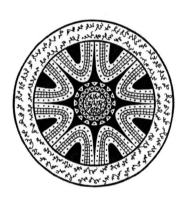

The ages have seen man, in various forms and stages of selfpity, piety and false humility, bargain with, appease and try to please and control his deities. The self-pity could only be assuaged by holier-than-thou self-importance. Self-pity has been a major obstacle to the discovery that what we have begged alms from has been ourselves.

Illumination 116

Self-importance has been a less painful illusion than self-pity. We clung to any perceived illusory advantage over others so that we did not have to acknowledge how lost we felt or how unreal the only life we knew was. When we did find the real and holy, we found ourselves in so much vastness that we constracted in angst. The way we

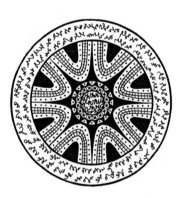

could stay in contraction was to enter into more and more doctrine and dogma, often at the point of overzealous bigotry.

The going back and forth in our silent times between the matrix and the formless place of True Beingness until we live from there is our trailblazing answer to this illusional dilemma.

Illumination 117

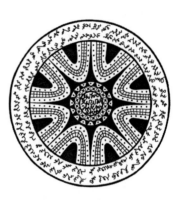

There is no real disagreement if we consider that there are no two beings in existence—only One. What then lies behind this seeming friction? It is the opportunity to step out of the unreal. There are no separate pieces within the One, nor can there be anything inharmonious with It. When we step out of the unreal we become like anti-matter within matter, cancelling out our own illusion. In this way we thin the veils and the illusory reality becomes a little less pervasive.

Illumination 118

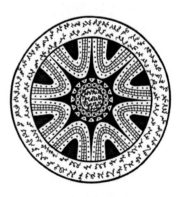

Much control has been exerted to create conformity among those we think should be our 'tribe'. Whether it is within family units, churches or communities, if there is sameness, one is accepted. If not there is even ostracism, or at best a withholding of approval.

The irony is that there is no sameness anywhere at any time. Every snowflake, flower or insect has its own individuality of appearance and expression of the One Life. The quest for sameness is illusory—it doesn't exist.

Illumination 119

The desires of the tribe, or controlling individuals, for conformity have created equally illusory tools — appropriateness and propriety.

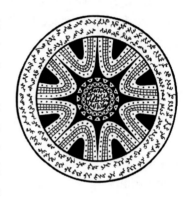

The self-appointed arbiters of what is 'decent' and 'fitting' and what is not have a mentor that pervasively spanned all created life — mind. Mind was also a self-appointed magistrate and absolute tyrant. It does not like nonconformity either, since it only feels comfortable with labels and predictability. Anything that challenges its control system is either ignored, attacked or ridiculed. Real Life cannot be lived within the illusion of a tribe.

Illumination 120

If nothing is out of place, how has an illusion-filled reality found its existence? There is an unreal delight being created like a pearl in an oyster. The timing of its fruition is vital as is the ability to develop strength and refinement created during its incubation period.

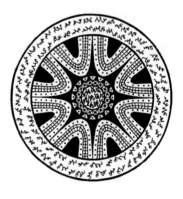

The illusion is both its embryonic sac and its timing mechanism. The illusional membranes will thin, allowing the birth at the correct developmental stage. The illusions within that are being discarded as obsolete are like the potter's clay falling away to reveal a refined creation.

Illumination 121

We think we are in control of ourselves but in truth, the body's life is so unreal, it is no more than a puppet on a string. Control is a myth, as is being 'out of control'.

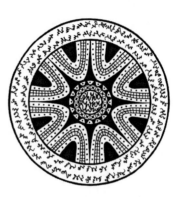

At times we feel so expanded it seems we are out of control of our lives. Even expanded, we are still within the One Being who runs our lives. It does not take our direct focus to run our lives.

Those who enter into Immortal Mastery know this principle well, for in this stage of human evolution speech, writing and living all occur within the total silence of mind.

Illumination 122

Thinking we are incomplete creates the illusion of achievement as a measuring stick of our worth. There is no achievement when there is no choice.

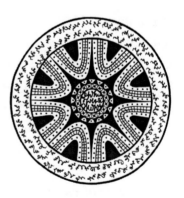

This matrix is like a dream—not really there. If within a dream the baker bakes good cookies, whose accomplishment is it? Is it the baker's or the dreamer's? It is the same way with our lives. We have come from the deeper levels of the dream into those more shallow. Yet we presume to look back and either cringe at our incompleteness or pat ourselves on the back for our accomplishments. But we have done neither. The Dreamer has been the one orchestrating the dream. The One Life has been pulling the strings.

Illumination 123

To fear we will encounter a void or a profoundly boring passivity when we enter the One Life is far from the truth. Multiple experiences of the One are required as we exit from the Dream for us to realize that we cannot see It, hear It or encounter It with any of our senses, even the inner ones. It must be experienced in Its boundlessness as we 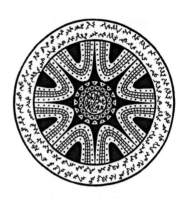 dissolve into It. It is our home, our being, ancient beyond any beginning. Yet we have forgotten how to participate in Our Being.

Realization will come back to us the more we see the realms of life and the more we shed the illusory spider web of form that overlays the perfection.

Illumination 124

Society has been seen as the supporter and creator of order, a surrogate parent to us. It has promised to provide us with amenities we believe we cannot live without in return for our obedience to its laws and rules. The manmade illusional structure of society is not needed to take care of us. We are governed by the One Life and do not need institu- 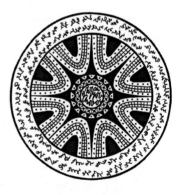 tions that promise us comfort, but then put us in bondage through debt and taxes. Our societies have generated enslavement to work and class-based structures. These illusions have become tyrants.

Illumination 125

The remnants of mind feel comfortable with structure. They thrive on clarity of meaning and labels. We see meaning in art, defining and analyzing it in the name of intellectualism and culture.

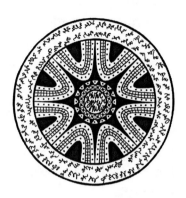

It is time to experience the purity of life directly, not through structured filters of analyses. Analysis is only another tool of mind, as is intellect. Life is a direct expression of the intangible, available to us only when we are open, spontaneous and trusting, like perpetual children. The promises of mind to provide us with a pristine world have proven untrustworthy.

Illumination 126

Eons of cataclysmic Earth changes have created fear that we may in some way be bringing them about. It also makes us feel we have lacked the power to prevent them. The Earth can be affected only by our One Life. At no time can our unreal forms affect the Earth's unreal form.

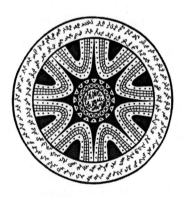

Earth too, has an internal, incorruptible part. Our interconnected, inseparable lives are also indivisibly one with the Earth. She is safe in the care of our Eternal Self.

Illumination 127

Accessing the shallow areas of life is not better than accessing it deeply. All its parts and levels are equally valid. Even if we have shallow experiential interactions, they can never be shallow if by that term we imply life is only partially accessed. Behind the illusory life of form is the vastness of the majestic All.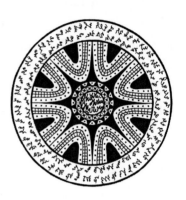

Through every seemingly insignificant action, the depths of the Infinite Life speak. Through the windows of our experiences the One sees Itself with delight.

Illumination 128

The illusion that wisdom exists implies that the indefinable can be labeled and there are static points in the Infinite's unfolding.

Life of form started in smaller 'boxes' of illusional containment. It is the wisdom of yesterday that got us to this point by breaking open one box after the other. The insights of obsolete 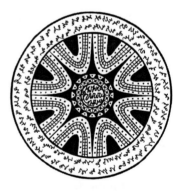 moments of dreaming cannot possibly apply to the present. They brought us to where we are, immediately outliving their usefulness as they broke down the walls.

It is time for us to leave behind our boxes of illusion. We are returning home to the Oneness and no wisdom with its static viewpoints can serve us there.

Illumination 129

The illusion of 'correct' or 'incorrect' implies that anything contrary to the real can exist, that life can be in opposition to itself, that opposites can exist. There can be nothing in existence that is out of place or un-whole or contrary to the Divine Perfection that permeates it all.

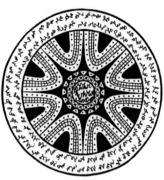

So much concern is given to making correct choices. Yet by manipulating our discernment and tastes, the One Life ensures that our choices never falter. They are always correct. We may lie back in the arms of the One Life and relax.

Illumination 130

What we perceive as obstacles, life turns into symbols of inclusion. The oppositions in our lives were never meant to be anything other than an intricate guidance system. The obstacle that suddenly arises on our path is the loving hand of the One Life directing us to go left or right, were we only to take the time to see. By seeing only the

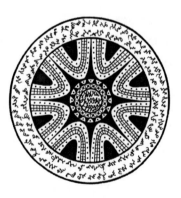

wall, we may not notice that when one door closes, another has just opened. The worst we can imagine is only a wave of the ocean. We will be carried up and over the wave. We are never alone.

Illumination 131

Fear exists that when we experience the vastness we may disassociate from life. The life we detach from is not real. We detach from the unreal without separation.

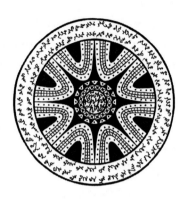

The truth behind this fear of not being able to run our lives is that we never really could do so, as evidenced by the flaws of manmade reality and the many stresses in our lives.

When our lives are surrendered to the Infinite, the fluid pattern becomes one of unfolding perfection—what it was always meant to be.

Illumination 132

The illusion of pain as inflicted by others or by life is a misrepresentation from our illusory belief systems. For the creation of individuated life for the delight of the One Being, an illusional fracturing that created illusory chambers occurred—much like the splitting of a cell. Those cells have been united as one illusion after another has been

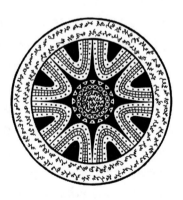

seen for what it is. The pain has been the pain of disconnection from our Real life of Oneness. This has been seen to be the case but, like the air that is as much inside the box as outside it, there has never really been separation, else this illusory world would not have animated life.

Illumination 133

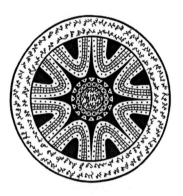

The sub-creations of our manmade world do not really exist. The real cannot be created by the unreal. The chair we sit on, the room we sleep in—nothing is actually there. It is just the result of mass hypnosis. The child in his playpen may try and build a bridge with his blocks but at the end of his playtime all will be removed and packed away.

The blocks we have been playing with are the building blocks of life, but ultimately they are unreal.

Illumination 134

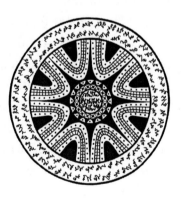

The mystical kingdoms are the reflections of the nuances of man. As such, they are as unreal as we are. All is being gathered back together. The 144 illuminations become one; no illusions have ever existed. The God-kingdoms are gathered into one kingdom. The Creation of the One Life will soon be ready to leave its incubator and become part of the nuances of Infinite Life. The mystical kingdoms' realities are getting ready to join with whence they came—the human kingdom.

Illumination 135

We nurture the illusion that we can teach and advise others, thinking we know what is best for them. Their past is illusory and cannot help determine the newness of the moment. To heal and save judges and divides. To acknowledge wholeness is to uplift all life by thinning the illusory veils that bind us. Each soul exists in the perfection 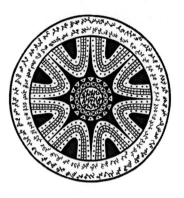 of his true Oneness. What can we ever teach anyone? This would only perpetuate the illusion of separation by enacting the illusion of relationship.

Illumination 136

Although we have fluidly tried to release and move beyond the obsolete memories of a past that does not exist, the damaging footprints of that past still mar the sands of our life with their imprints. This is because imagined creations are not able to change and keep pace as fluidly as the unfolding of Infinite Life.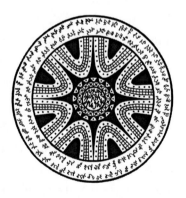

If we are not created as a separate creation but as an everchanging impression of the unfolding nuances of the One Life, there are no lasting impressions. This is what we have truly always been. Lasting impressions have never been a reality.

Illumination 137

The imagined momentary spot called Creation that formed within the Infinite's boundless unfolding has taken on a life of its own, even though it is unreal. There is no place where the Infinite is not and Its presence permeates even the illusory portion of Its Being where this imagined creation took place, thereby enlivening it.

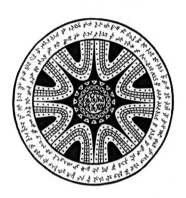

Anything the One Life creates or that is not, is a baser addition that cannot exist. Nothing should ever be created; it would detract from the whole and create space. What then are you and I as the One Life? We are beginningless and real as impressions of the unfolding nuances of the Infinite.

Illumination 138

Within the true Beingness we are, there are no polarities, no rest or activity, no beingness and doingness. In desiring to experience interaction with the imagined creation, the four levels of dreaming came into being. The Infinite created a dream body and entered into the dream with Its illusory body in the illusion of relationship.

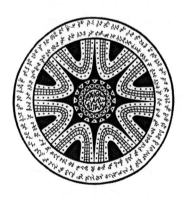

Within the moment formed by the 'pulse' or 'pop' in the timelessness of Infinite Life, all eons of existence occurred. Like an entire book contained on microfilm in the dot of the letter 'i', all life has occurred within the illusion of the moment. It is impossible for dreaming or sleep to occur. It is not possible for a moment to be created in Infinite Life.

Illumination 139

The definition of illusion is the desire for the unreal to be real. The tools illusion created to fulfill its desire are fantasy, daydreaming and imagination. These three tools gave rise to the three directions of the above, the below and the within. In turn, the first three stages of linear time and illusory creation began.

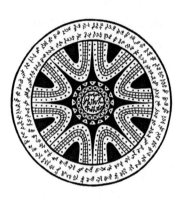

The Infinite has no actual movement, but unfolding, alternating impressions. The One Life creates the impressions of form for its delight—not as static shape but fluid boundary-less impressions.

Illumination 140

The illusory way in which we see events unfold within the illusion-based senses of form creates the impressions of continuity and repetitiveness. The factor of the illusion of the moment contributes to this. Imagine the Infinite beingness in unfolding fluidity. Imagine that within it a 'pop' happens. The pop has just created a moment,

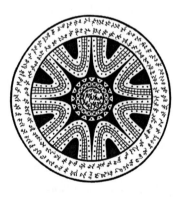

because there was a time it occurred and a time it did not. A moment in a place of no-time is an anomaly; something that does not belong. The result is that, like a rubber ball thrown on the floor, it seems to bounce over and over again. This gives the impression of continuity but in fact it's the same moment repeating. Because you imagined it, it was never really there.

Illumination 141

There can be no over-focus because there is no reference point. There can be no addiction because the One Life can never abandon Itself. The unreal cannot have influence of any kind in seeming desirable or indispensible or real to the One Life, for it does not exist.

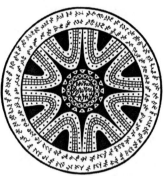

When the first pulse within the Infinite became important as something new or attractive, illusion was seemingly born. Yet none of this is real or has ever existed.

Mind was formed by the hypnotic effect of the unreal and the attraction it had for the One life. Thus, one illusion begat another.

Illumination 142

A heartbeat, like a single pulse, was imagined within the One Life. But because there is no time, it set that moment apart from the no-time. The effect of having a momentary heartbeat was that it repeated itself over and over, like a record that has gotten stuck. The result was that a heartbeat was born. This is extremely confusing

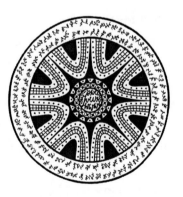

and contradictory. It defined a space where it could be most strongly heard or felt. This area could be defined as a heart. Further out from what now became an illusory reference point, the area that was still affected by the heartbeat became a body. The illusion that anything new can be created, such as a pulse, implies that there is something the Infinite does not know—an impossibility since there is nothing beyond the One Life.

Illumination 143

As more attention was given to the heartbeat, it was able to receive more and more and became receptive. Femininity was born as an illusion. The imbalance this created generated a lightning flash. The masculine polarity was formed. The split of masculine and feminine from the androgynous One Life gave duality as an illusion.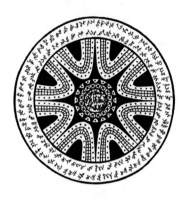
The heart received an electrical shock that split it into four ventricles. Four spaces were created and the four directions were born.

By never having encountered anything unreal before—because in fact it did not exist—the Infinite assumed everything to be real. Now the illusion of seeking to understand the unreal was formed.

Illumination 144

The seeming splitting created many illusions: that loss or damage could occur and that something could occur outside the One's control. There were many questions that arose and the act of questioning created density of form as it became more real and solid from focusing on it. The created illusional realities we have been in are the result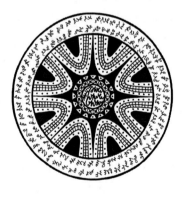
of the Infinite 'fixing' the fracturing of the heart it had formed. Like a wound that develops thick and hard scar tissue, life became dense where the fracturing had occurred.

The embodiment of the part of the Infinite that was focusing on it was drawn into the scar tissue or dense creations by Its questions and mind became an illusory tool for finding the way out of the web of illusion.

Saradesi Satva Yoga Postures

The Postures

The purpose of Saradesi Satva Yoga's postures is to remove linear time—the primary cause of aging and decay. In removing the opposites of movement and stillness by balancing them, we cancel them out to reveal a state of eternal rejuvenation.[1]

Saradesi Satva Yoga alternates movement and stillness. The movement expresses, the stillness listens. The movements are slow and deliberate like those found in the more feminine styles of martial arts. This type of movement can best be described as 'stillness within movement'. During the motionless postures, the mind becomes completely silent. The motions too are done mindlessly as the depth of our being expresses.

The moving postures express the feeling of verses in *The Poetry of Dreaming*[2]. Movements are done as an intuitive response of the body to experiencing the dream poetry. (The verses given with this yoga are but examples of a few such verses and they can be supplemented with others from *The Poetry of Dreaming*.) The motionless postures enter into the feelings evoked by the images. Immersing the self into the still postures, the practitioner enters the feeling of the poetic verse while doing the guided posture. The Saradesi yoga sound elixirs are played throughout the yoga.

THE POETRY OF DREAMING
Excerpted From Shrihat Satva Yoga

Cosmic cycles of life fall into two categories: those that can be called the ascension cycles and those that are called the descension cycles.

---

1 Highly recommended reading: *Secrets of Rejuvenation* by Almine.
2 See *Labyrinth of the Moon* for Poetry of Dreaming.

83

There are 12 electrical, masculine, light-based cycles; these are the ascension cycles. Likewise there are 12 cycles of a feminine, magnetic, frequency-based nature. Each of these has been repeated many times by all creatures as incarnation cycles.

The unresolved issues of those cycles, such as old belief systems, memories of pain and other distorted emotions are presented for resolution in dreams. There are 24 depths of dreaming, with the 12 more shallow ones communicating to us through dream symbols. The 12 deepest dream states are the feminine, non-cognitive states that cannot be interpreted through dream symbols and produce what to us seems like a deep, dreamless sleep. They speak to us through art and the Poetry of Dreaming.

This unique poetry communicates through omissions—that which is not said—imparting multiple depths of meaning revealing themselves as feelings and qualities. Although the Poetry of Dreaming uses literary devices such as assonance, alliteration, personification and sustained epithets, their use has profound purpose that transcends the obvious. The same applies to the use of adjectives in this type of poetry.

Its concise but powerful descriptive quality is reminiscent of the poetic form called Haiku, but whereas Haiku is bound by a rigid structure, the Poetry of Dreaming is not. Haiku provides the essence of simplicity that lies within the complexity of appearances. The Poetry of Dreaming whispers, through its rich imagery, of the primordial origins of the moment.

... The Poetry of Dreaming is used to open non-cognitive communication with the deeper states of dreaming. This allows the issues of very old cycles of life to come to the surface for cancellation.

... It is recommended that the student meditate on the concept associated with the posture for ten to fifteen minutes preparatory to commencing the yoga session.

... The music for this purpose is unique and irreplaceable because it is sung in the Solfeggio scale. This is the scale used for Gregorian chants until it was banned by the Catholic Church in the early Middle Ages. Its effect of liberating the listener from belief systems is profound.

The method is simple. The student reads the verse, empties his or her mind through entering a meditative state, and simply observes any images that arise and the subtle feelings they evoke.

... At no time should analysis be used. The more empty the mind, the more successful the non-cognitive communication from the deep psyche can be. Capturing in writing the images that arise can be helpful. Different students may receive communications in different forms.

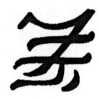

MOVEMENT 1

The sun sets. Tree branches blacken against the night sky like flotsam adrift in an endless sea. The frog welcomes the evening star.

> With this movement, release belief systems around the aging of the body and all associations of a specific age. Remembering the freedom of childhood and how comfortable we felt with the body and its movements will help to free up the stuck patterns of these belief systems in the body.

Suggested Interpretations
- Feel the endlessness of life's alternating cycles. As one closes, another begins. Viewed from a timeless perspective, all is one; all happens at the same time.

- The essence of the tree is eternal, yet its form fluidly seems to change with the coming of the night. In the endless contradiction of existence, the tree exists in changeless change.
- The frog and the star are interacting within the interconnectedness of life. One gives joy, the other appreciation. Size is nothing to the Infinite and all play a significant part.

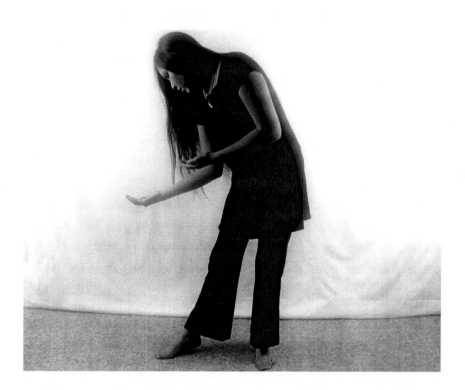

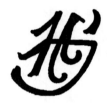

SEATED POSTURE 1

> The hand and eye movements of this posture are
> designed to release programs of aging held in the heart
> center, brain and behind the eyes. The breathing pattern
> associated with these movements releases confining
> beliefs that have stunted self-expression in the lungs.

The Posture

With your legs stretched in front of you, sit with your spine straight,
feet about six inches apart. Your chin is level as you look straight
ahead. With arms straight and parallel to your sides, rest your hands
on the floor and point them outward, pointing away from the body.

The Method

- Breathe in deeply through the nose. As you breathe, lift the arms
  —still parallel to the sides at shoulder height—and gently raise
  the head to look at the ceiling.
- With hands still pointing sideways, raise the arms only to shoulder height.
- Return to the starting position for this posture as you breathe out
  through the mouth.

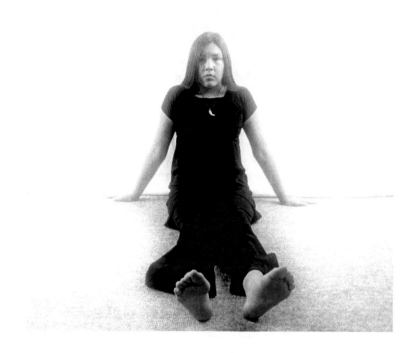

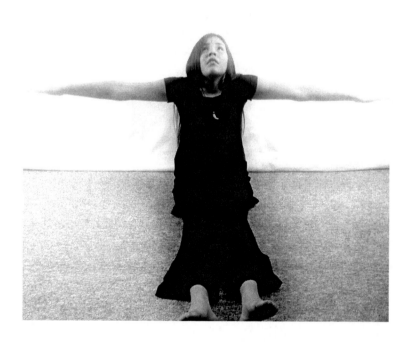

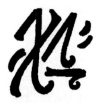

MOVEMENT 2

In the firelight's glow the aging Labrador sleeps on his well-worn blanket. His muscles twitch as he chases a rabbit across the moonlit field.

Allow your movements to express opposites and gradually feel these opposites combine into a harmonious state of oneness. The movement and posture is designed specifically to release the illusional belief that the body and soul are separate. Immortal beings have successfully managed through inner integration to end the polarity of life and death.

Suggested Interpretations
- When comfort is valued over discomfort, the outer life grows and the inner life wanes. When both are equally embraced, the inner and outer worlds merge in mystical union.
- The verse suggests that the dream is really being experienced by the dog and the rabbit; that dreaming and awakening are one.
- Clinging to the familiar, as to a well-worn blanket, creates a rut that limits resources and causes bodily aging. It leaves the body behind. Transcending the limitation of mortality rejuvenates.

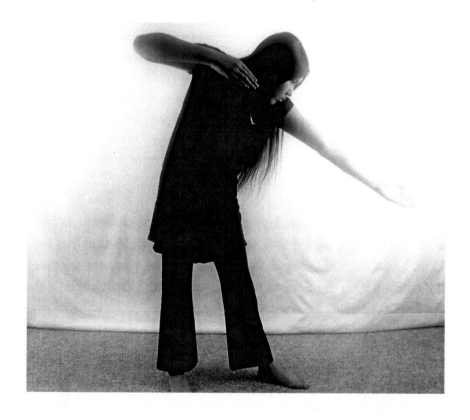

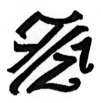

SEATED POSTURE 2

Designed to allow the programs of life and death to be dissolved and the knowingness of the reality of eternal life to surface. During this posture allow the feeling of infinity, of having no beginning or end, to permeate the body.

The Posture

Sit with the spine straight, legs apart. The legs are straight and form a 'V' shape. Keeping the back straight and the chin level as you face ahead, lean slightly forward. With arms straight, place the palms of the hands flat on the floor in front of you about 8 inches apart with the fingers pointing forward.

The Method

- Take a deep breath in through the nose while remaining in the original position.
- Breathe out through the mouth while lowering your chin onto your chest and moving your hands forward as far as is comfortable. Keep your back straight.
- Move back to the original position while breathing in through the nose.

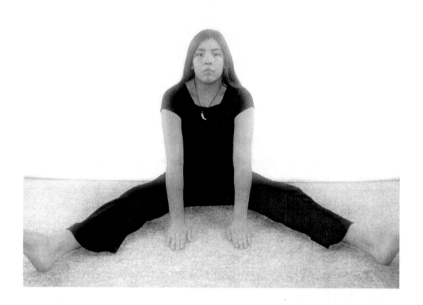

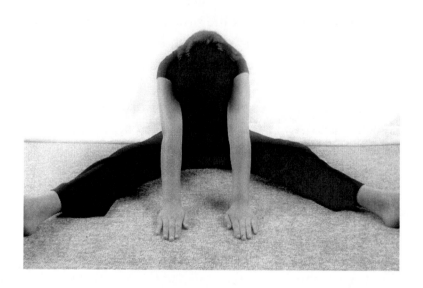

MOVEMENT 3

Lace curtains flutter in the night breeze. The moon reaches with
tender fingers to stroke the downy cheek of the sleeping child.

> The combination of the posture and movement is
> designed to bring resolution to the illusion of movement
> and stillness. Since all happens at once, movement
> can be regarded as layers of stillness that have been
> separate from one another. Feel the stillness within the
> movements you create.

Suggested Interpretations

- Consider the lightness of the scenario; the carefree trust of a well-loved child who knows that life sustains him; the weightlessness and fluid dance of curtains and wind. Fluid perspective and perceptional changes are the hallmarks of mastery.
- Beauty is not what it seems—a flat, two-dimensional image that social learning validates. It is the fleeting and fluid interaction of elements of existence that evoke the deep peace and rapture of the unfolding majesty of existence.

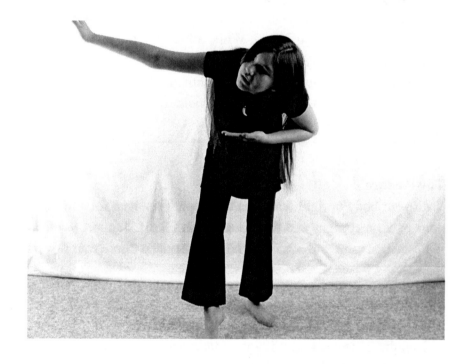

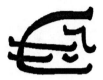

SEATED POSTURE 3

An empowered being knows him or herself to be the
center of their universe—the pivot point that can change
all by changing ourselves. While all moves, the pivot
point is in silence. During this posture allow the body's
borders to dissolve into its environment, that the illusion
of the still reference point might yield to movement
within stillness.

The Posture

With your body upright, kneel on the floor. Then lean forward until
your back is straight and horizontal to the floor. Support yourself
with straight arms and with your hands flat on the floor. Your fingers
are pointed forward.

The Method

- Sit with the back straight, face looking forward.
- Breathe in deeply, dropping your face down onto your chest and,
  arching your back upwards, make it as round as possible. Breathe
  in through the nose.
- Sigh the breath out slowly through the mouth while sagging the
  chest downward and raising your head to face forward.
- Repeat.

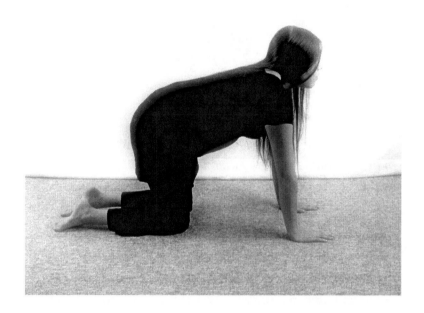

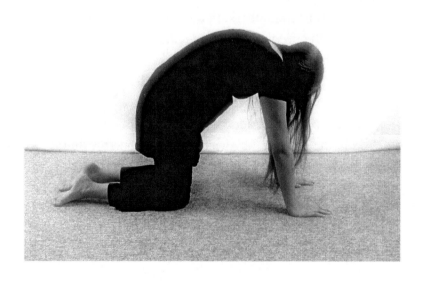

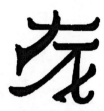

MOVEMENT 4

In the soil made rich by fallen leaves, the slumbering acorn awakes to the rustle of Spring. A blue jay builds a nest in the great oak tree.

> Allow your body to feel the complete freedom of changelessly changing like an eternal ocean. There is no death, nor life, for whatever is real does not have an opposite. There is just the timeless existence of eternal life.

Suggested Interpretations
- In man the Infinite slumbers; in the Infinite man awakes.
- The acorn is the product of the tree and the tree is the product of the acorn. The cycle of life never ends.
- Without beginning or end, our form fluidly changing, we enter timelessness.
- That which we judge as unconsciousness is but the slumbering of the seed in the ground. Its awakening is in perfect timing. There is only perfection.

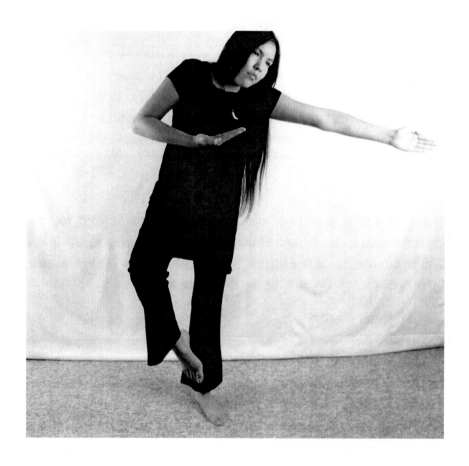

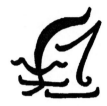

SEATED POSTURE 4

Contemplate an island in an ocean and the statement
that the ocean is in the island and the island is in the
ocean. Existence is within you and you are within
existence. Feel this until you embody spaceless space.

Posture

Sit upright with your back straight and the soles of your feet together as you face forward. Hold your knees with your hands under
and to the outside of the knees. Your palms will be facing upward,
your head facing forward. Grasp the knees firmly.

The Method

- Breathe in through the nose while raising your shoulders level
  with your ears.
- Slowly breathe out through your mouth as you lower your shoulders. Lower your chin onto your chest.
- With the next in-breath, raise the chin and face outward as you
  raise the shoulders again.
- Repeat.

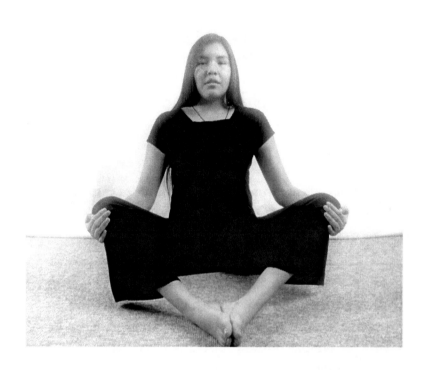

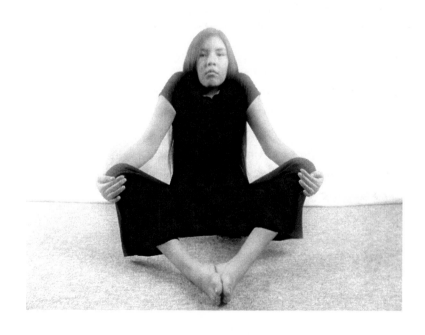

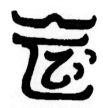

MOVEMENT 5

*The snow geese watch the clouds move to shroud the
hoary-headed mountains. Inspired by the sight, they leave
as one on their southward journey.*

Allow all self-consciousness and self-reflection to melt
away through your movements. Like a child at play
become the wind and the clouds, the rain and the earth.
Be fully present within yourself as you release self-
consciousness, belief systems of acceptable standards,
and personal identities—becoming as free as the wind.

Suggested Interpretations
- In watching for the trigger events in our life, we need not let hardship steer our course. Beauty and inspiration can be the way-showers.
- Sensitivity to our environment makes truth—the next step in the unfolding dance of existence—self-evident. The concept of personal opinion becomes obsolete.

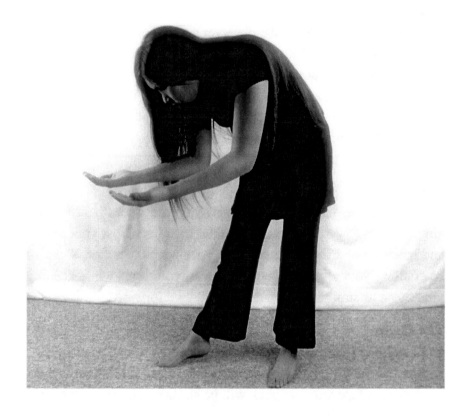

SEATED POSTURE 5

Allow yourself to be the observer and the observed.
Be fully present with your posture but allow your
awareness to observe it the way your hands enclose
the priceless treasure of a moving butterfly. We are the
music and the musician, the actor and the playwright.
Let all identity with roles melt away.

The Posture

Begin by sitting with your spine straight, your knees bent and facing upwards towards the ceiling, ankles together. Cross your ankles and reach around the knees to clasp your hands together. You will be cradling your slightly opened knees in your arms while keeping your spine as straight as possible as you face forward.

The Method

- Remaining in the position, breathe in deeply through the nose.
- Breathe out slowly while dropping the head and slumping the shoulders forward. The back will be slightly rounded as the head and shoulders relax forward.
- On the in-breath, resume the original position by raising the head and straightening the spine.
- Repeat.

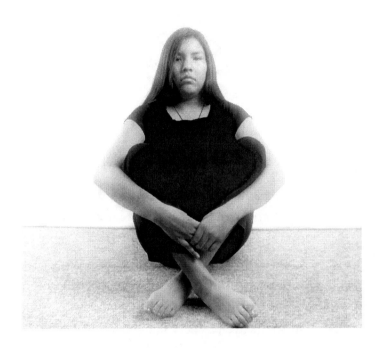

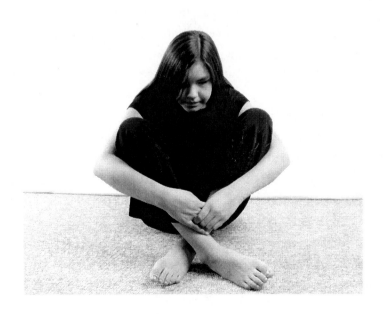

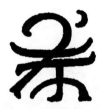

MOVEMENT 6

Night bells ring from the monastery, singing the sleepy town to rest. Sleigh bells, like tinkling laughter, answer from a snowy field.

Feel the timelessness of life, like a beating heart creating its cyclical ages like the inbreath and the outbreath of God. You are its cycles and when the inbreath and outbreath become one, eternal life flourishes. Eternal existence flourishes and life and death are no more. You are the beating of the swallow's wings, the mighty ocean that beats against the shore, you are the inbreath and outbreath of Infinite existence. Release the belief systems of size and shape and identity.

Suggested Interpretations

- The monastery bells are stationary and reliable; something that can be depended upon to announce that all is well. Yet their sound fluidly moves. All our actions have consequences that ripple throughout existence.
- The sleigh bells do not take themselves seriously. They do not have the honored respect of many, but though unrecognized and unacclaimed, they bring merriment and lightheartedness—the counterpart in the symphony of bells on a snowy night.

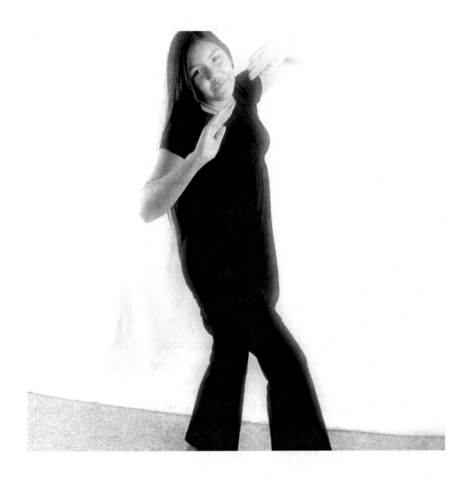

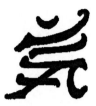

SEATED POSTURE 6

> Become a portal of life, all flows through you. There
> is no difference between in and out, no directions and
> no beginning or end. Nothing exists without that does
> not exist within. Allow the fluid sovereignty of such an
> existence to be felt in every cell of your body.

The Posture

Kneel and place your hands flat on the floor in front of you, shoulder-width apart. Sit back on your haunches as far as is comfortable while facing forward.

The Method

- The body posture is maintained throughout in a relaxed stretch.
- With every in-breath, the head faces forward, the chin parallel to the floor. Breathe in through the nose.
- With every out-breath, slowly lower the chin to the chest. Breathe out through the mouth.
- Repeat in a slow, rhythmic way.

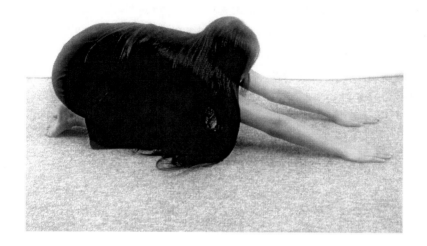

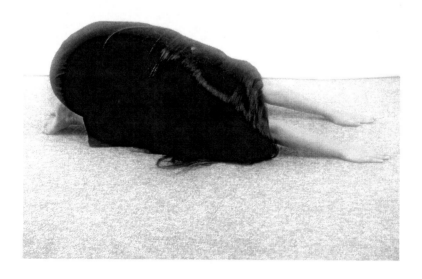

CLOSING

We live in a time of fulfillment of great prophecies from ancient origins. We are living, according to those prophecies, during a time when all will overcome the causes of aging and decay; when resources will again be mastered that can sustain continual rejuvenation. This will begin with just a few who will dare to challenge belief systems and mortal boundaries. They will stand as shining examples until all realize that eternal rejuvenation is the birthright of man.

May this day be now.

Almine

Appendix I

NOTES FOR TEACHERS

The yoga may be taught to others if the practitioner has become proficient in its practices. No other training is needed because its effectiveness is inherent in its components.

Appendix II

LIABILITY DISCLAIMER

Any liability, loss, damage or injury in connection with the use of this yoga and its instruction, including but not limited to any performance of the yoga, is expressly disclaimed by Spiritual Journeys, LLC and/or Almine.

Many have subluxations and misalignments in the neck. Seeking chiropractic treatment prior to attempting Saradesi Satva Yoga may be beneficial. The neck extensions and movements of Saradesi Satva Yoga should be done gently and with care not to strain the neck.

Yoga is not intended to diagnose illness or to constitute medical advice or treatment. Any student whose medical condition, including pregnancy or any other health-related condition that may affect performance of the yoga, is advised to consult with a physician or other qualified health provider prior to the start of this program and obtain approval to participate in the yoga.

Other Yoga Products by Almine

Irash Satva Yoga
Shrihat Satva Yoga
Labyrinth of the Moon
The Abundant Life

Other Books By Almine

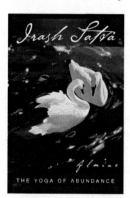

Irash Satva Yoga

Yoga, as a spiritual and physical discipline has been practiced in many variations by masters and novices for countless years and is universally accepted as one of the most effective development tools ever created.

Man's physical form in its original state was meant to be self-purifying, self-regenerating and self-transfiguring. Through pristine living and total surrender, it was possible to open gates in the body that would allow life to permeate and lfow through it; indefinitely sustaining it.

In IRASH SATVA YOGA, received by Almine from the Angelic Kingdom, this ancient methodology is exponentially expanded and enhanced by incorporating the alchemies of sound and frequency.

Using easily mastered postures paired with music from Cosmic Sources created specifically for each, the 144 cardinal gates in the mind and body are opened and cleansed of their dross and debris, allowing the practitioner to tap into the abundance of the One Life.

Published: 2010, 94 pages, soft cover, 6 × 9, $24.95; ISBN: 978-1-934070-95-6

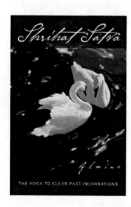

Shrihat Satva Yoga

The human body is unique in that it is an exact microcosm of the macrocosm of created life. There are 12 points along the right, masculine side of the body and the same number on the left side. These are microcosmic replicas of the macrocosmic cycles of life.

The yoga postures are designed to open and remove the debris from these points – the gates of dreaming. This will occur physically through the postures and the music. Dissolving debris also occurs by way of dreaming (triggered by the breathing and eye movements), releasing past issues that caused the blockages in the points.

Published: 2010, 108 pages, soft cover, 6 × 9, $34.95; ISBN: 978-1-934070-15-4

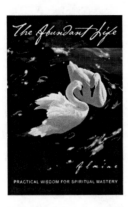

The Abundant Life

By popular demand, the profound words of wisdom that have changed the lives of more than 20,000 daily Twitter followers, communicating in multiple languages, have been compiled into book form.

Three hundred aphorisms and mandalas from the Seer Almine will delight and inspire her growing global audience.

Published: 2010, 188 pages, soft cover, 6 × 9, $19.95; ISBN: 978-1-934070-20-8

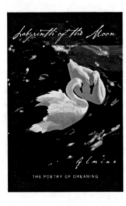

Labyrinth of the Moon

The book contains 144 verses of the Poetry of Dreaming and extensive lists of the interpretation of dream symbols. It is a valuable tool for opening up the deeper dream-states' communications, promoting the healing of the psyche, the body and facilitating the balance of the Inner Child and other sub-personalities.

Designed to release the hold of past incarnational cycles, it is an essential companion for practitioners of Shrihat and Saradesi Satva Yoga.

Published: 2010, 188 pages, soft cover, 6 × 9, $19.95; ISBN: 978-1-934070-10-9

Almine is the author of many other books.
All are available on
www.spiritualjourneys.com

LaVergne, TN USA
06 April 2011
223003LV00004B/7/P